TEST
AND
GROW
HEALTHY

TEST AND GROW HEALTHY

How You Can Turn Your Body into a Health-Building Machine

SANFORD "BUDDY" FRUMKER, D.D.S.

Health Associates, Inc.
CLEVELAND, OHIO

This Book is Dedicated to
the Memory of
Dr. Richard Broeringmeyer

With never ending gratitude for his great wisdom,
for his incredible guidance, and for the miracle of health
he made available to so many!

And to

All of our students who experience disease—and the
achievement of health—as a never ending challenge
and a continual opportunity for greater self-growth
and self-empowerment.

To My Wonderful Family

With a heart full of love and overflowing appreciation to:

Beatrice, my magnificent, fantastic, and always supportive
wife of 53 years!

And to:

Shelley, Elaine, and Loren, my three children;

Bill, Thor, and Marcy, their spouses;

Marissa, Michael, Emily, and Lindsay my four grandchil-
dren; for the incredible joy and wonder they have endlessly
added to my life!

And deep thanks to:

Joan Tilow, Doris Palmer, and Laurie Regal, who have shared
the 40 plus years of my practice so as to not only develop
a wonderful practice, but for us to mutually develop and
enhance each other.

HOW TO CONTACT THE AUTHOR

A Biohealth practitioner and professional spearker, Dr. Sanford "Buddy" Frumker was an associate of Dr. Richard Broeringmeyer from 1983 until Dr. Broeringmeyer's untimely death in 1991. Together they presented many one-day workshops.

Since then, Dr. Frumker has carried on and greatly expanded the workshops.

Dr. Frumker teaches participants the Biohealth Program step-by-step. Attendees not only learn how to do the Biohealth Program, they discover a great deal about their own health and their own body.

To arrange a one-day workshop or a speaking engagement, contact:

Dr. Sanford Frumker
1731 Wrenford Road
Cleveland, OH 44121
Phone and fax: 216-382-3317

CONTENTS

Preface. ix

Introduction: *Why This Book Had to Be Written* 1

Chapter 1 ● Five Medical Myths That Make
Biohealth a Necessity for You. 11

Chapter 2 ● The Biohealth System—Adventures
in the Body Electric 23

Chapter 3 ● The Universe You Live In—What Is It?
Why Is It? Where Is It Now?
Where Is It Going? 43

Chapter 4 ● Growing Younger as You Become
Older—How Your Body Functions 57

Chapter 5 ● The Biohealth System—
Test and Grow Healthy! 69

Chapter 6 ● What Is Magnetism? 79

Chapter 7 ● The Hydrogen Ion and pH. 91

Chapter 8 ● How Cellular Change Leads
to Malfunction and Disease 97

Chapter 9 ● The Biohealth Personality 103

Chapter 10 ● Creating Health That Lasts—
How to Use Magnetic Testing
to Achieve Energy Balance 111

Chapter 11 ● The Basic Magnetic Examination 131

Chapter 12 ● The Fundamentals—How to Correct
Imbalances and Maintain Biohealth . . . 157

Chapter 13 ● Some Important Odds and Ends—
Healthy Foods and Disease Patterns . . 193

Chapter 14 ● Three Deadly Problems—
Cancer, Heart Disease and Pain 203

Chapter 15 ● You Do Not Have the Right to Be Sick! . . 231

Appendix A: *Supplies* 241

Appendix B: *Health Services* 245

Appendix C: *Reading List* 247

Index 253

PREFACE

The Biohealth System answers two of the most vital questions in your life:

What can you do *right now* to achieve your highest level of health?

What can you then do to maintain that highest level of health?

The answers to these questions are so important because when your body is functioning correctly and maintaining its highest level of health, the rest of your life tends to fall in line.

No one is destined to live a carefree, unchallenged life but true health gives you the opportunity to make the most out of your life and your potential while dealing effectively with the many stresses of day-to-day living.

Wouldn't it be wonderful if you had a health program that would be under your control and by which you could achieve your highest level of health? Such a program is now available. It is called the Biohealth System. You learn how to do this program not by reading about it but by doing it. As you work through this book, you will achieve your highest level of health.

Your first step is to accurately test how healthy you are. The next step is to determine the specific health program needed to bring you to your best level of health. Then you follow the program, continuously testing it to be sure it is moving you to higher levels of health.

A key to the Biohealth Program is testing. Everything you do, every step you take, is tested to be sure it is moving you toward higher health. *You do not guess or hope in the Biohealth Program; you test and know.* The Biohealth System uses magnetic testing, a "window" through which you look into your own body and "see" exactly what is going on. After you achieve health, you monitor it so you know exactly how to stay healthy. Every step of the Biohealth Program is monitored by magnetic testing, in which you will become an expert.

If the above sounds challenging and exciting to you, you are a prime candidate for the Biohealth System. You will rapidly learn that while you may use professional help, *only you can do the testing that is required for you to reach and maintain your highest level of health.*

Unlike other approaches to health, the Biohealth System doesn't wait for disease to come and then cure it. Its focus is on creating health now. Why? The answer is quite simple: When your body produces health you become immune to disease. Health and disease do not exist in the same body at the same time. When you have disease or illness, you do not have health. When you have health (or more accurately "Biohealth") you do not have disease.

The goal of Biohealth is to get you healthy and keep you healthy because as long as you are healthy, you will be immune to disease. Under the Biohealth System, the whole focus of health care changes from the negative to the positive. Instead of focusing on disease and its frightening possibilities you focus on the exciting potentials offered to you by health. Rather than fighting disease, you promote health.

The Single Most Important Health Fact You Will Ever Learn

When you begin the Biohealth Program, you will learn the most important single fact for having a lifetime of health: *Your best source of health comes from* within *your body, not from* outside *your body!*

The healing and health produced by the Biohealth Program comes from within your own body! In this way, Biohealth improves life. It lengthens life. You achieve increased energy and vitality. You avoid sickness and suffering because you become immune to disease.

Aging becomes more a matter for the calendar than biology.

You live to your full potential.

You enjoy life to its fullest.

You achieve whole body health.

Benefits of the Biohealth System

Following are just a few of the benefits the Biohealth System provides:

• It saves time. Time is a very limited and valuable commodity in our busy lives. The Biohealth System allows you to avoid becoming a hostage to our society's bureaucratic, inefficient medical system. You avoid lengthy office visits, procedures and hours spent in waiting rooms. And with Biohealth you *immediately* know the results of your tests.

• It saves money. The Biohealth System is very inexpensive.

• It empowers you. The Biohealth System puts your health in your hands. Your own body—not doctors—not drugs—replaces diseases with health. While the skill and experience of doctors remain important, and medications may be important, you are no longer dependent on them. The Biohealth System lets you know when, where and how health professionals and drugs should be used and gives you a way to evaluate how effective they are in helping you. You break out of the disease industry prison. You know what is working and what is not and thus gain control of your health and life.

- It is not invasive. There are no needles or intrusive and painful procedures.

- It does no harm. There are no dangerous side effects to the Biohealth System.

- It is not localized. You don't focus on body parts or putting out disease fires as they flare up. You focus on the whole body.

- It restores healthy function. Rather than fighting the symptoms and diseases, Biohealth goes straight to the source of ill health. Traditional therapy substitutes drugs and technology for health. With Biohealth you restore healthy functions, you achieve health and you do not need drugs. The Biohealth System is not a substitute health. It uses the tremendous powers of your own body to achieve total health.

- It is 100 percent natural.

- It is painless.

- It is easy and convenient. All the instruction you need to begin the program is contained in this book.

- It restores the health-producing powers of your own body. It restores them not only temporarily, but for your lifetime. The Biohealth Program puts you in communication with your own body, and *your own body* tells you what to do!

Most importantly, there are no questions about the effectiveness of the Biohealth System. Why? Because you test it.

Why This Book Had to Be Written

To be alive, only to be alive, may I never forget the privilege of that!

—Llewelyn Powys, *Skin for Skin*

My background is in traditional dental training. I began as a dentist specializing in periodontics (the treatment of gum tissue), occlusion (treatment of bite) and TMJ (temporomandibular joint dysfunction—or jaw pain). I was a board-certified periodontist in the Cleveland area. I wrote a textbook on occlusal treatment, won my share of dental honors and taught at Case Western Reserve Dental School in Cleveland where I served as an associate clinical professor for 42 years.

But dentistry was never enough for me. Soon after I began my career I found myself being drawn to other fields of health care that extended well beyond the confines of teeth and gum tissue. I sought out experts in physical medicine, nutrition, bioelectromagnetic energy and other fields and learned everything I could.

In 1983, I heard about the work of Dr. Richard Broeringmeyer. Dr. Broeringmeyer had three doctoral degrees. He was a

1

chiropractor with a DC, he had a DN in naturopathy (the treatment of disease through natural means) and a PhD in nutrition. He used his studies, experience and unique perspective to perfect a one-of-a-kind total health program that was achieving amazing results. I attended a workshop in North Carolina and was very impressed. After the workshop was over, I asked Dr. Broeringmeyer and his wife Mary to join me for dinner.

It was a fateful night. We immediately hit it off and found much common ground. By the time dinner was over Dr. Broeringmeyer and I had agreed to work together. After collaborating for two marvelous years we became partners in 1985, working closely together until his death in 1991.

How Dr. Broeringmeyer Forever Changed My Life

Dr. Broeringmeyer had developed a unique approach to health. *He did not believe any doctor in the world could influence a patient as well as the patient's own body could.* He despised the word "patient" because to him patients were people who felt helpless and inferior, agreeing to turn their health completely over to trained professionals who were far superior.

Richard believed that, to get well and reach his or her highest level of health, a "patient" had to communicate with and understand his or her own body. People must play a *major role* in their own health program.

This was a much different approach than I'd seen with any other health professional. They believed themselves to be the "experts" and that health could come only through their great knowledge and expertise. The "patient" had nothing to do with his or her own health. It was all up to the doctor.

Richard took great exception to this. He pointed out that the original meaning of the term "doctor" was "teacher." He claimed he did not have "patients" but "students." And he worked with them not as a superior (doctor) to an inferior (patient) but as a teacher to a student. His highest goal was for these "stu-

2

dents" to graduate from his workshops and ultimately become students of the greatest teacher of all—their own bodies.

Likewise, Dr. Broeringmeyer has some unique ideas about illness. His main focus was not on disease. It was on achieving health. He believed that disease and health were mutually exclusive. They could not coexist in the same body at the same time. By attaining health, you could make your body virtually immune to disease. Rather than declaring war on disease and fighting it, Dr. Broeringmeyer and his students replaced disease with health.

He also believed that total health involved much more than an occasional visit to the doctor when you didn't feel well. It was a full-time job. And a dynamic, ever-changing one. As we grow older, our health needs change. As stress in our life comes and goes, our health needs are constantly changing and require continual updating and adjustment. Dr. Broeringmeyer believed that, since you were the only person who lives with yourself 24 hours a day, you were the only one capable of maintain your health. The role of the doctor in Richard's mind was not so much to cure disease as it was to continually guide and update his or her students so they had the knowledge and abilities to take responsibility for their own health.

How Dr. Broeringmeyer Turned Sick "Patients" Into Healthy "Students"

Dr. Broeringmeyer found that it usually took one day to give a "patient" the basic knowledge and skills to become a successful "student." He also found that the best way to teach came through interaction. Therefore, rather than seeing people individually, he provided one-day workshops for his students. He called these Biohealth Workshops and I gave many of these workshops with Dr. Broeringmeyer.

Usually there were 25 to 30 people at each workshop. About one-quarter were health professionals wanting to learn Dr. Broeringmeyer's technique. A very few were people who wanted

3

to learn about health. The rest, the large majority, were people who had serious disease. Most had terminal cancer and had been given a short life expectancy by their doctors. They came to the workshops out of desperation.

The morning portion of the workshop consisted of lecture, discussion and demonstration. In the afternoon, everyone paired up and performed Biohealth techniques on each other. They learned by doing, under our watchful eyes. By the end of the day they had the knowledge and skills necessary to begin their own Biohealth Program.

If the student had a doctor or health professional we urged that he or she be added to our team. Biohealth is not an exclusive activity. Dr. Broeringmeyer welcomed and acknowledged the worth of skills from other health professionals. With Biohealth training the student was able to evaluate the care being given to them by their doctor or other health professional. We always welcomed anyone who could add to our knowledge and make our program more effective.

To continue to guide and help our students, Dr. Broeringmeyer had a toll-free telephone number so our students could call in and give us their progress and test readings, and we could give them our guidance. We became true doctors, teachers working at an eye-to-eye level with our students as equals.

This was an experience that forever changed my life. Usually, in 6 to 12 months, we would return to a city to give another workshop. We'd see the same people who, 6 to 12 months earlier, had come to our workshops with terminal cancer and were now cancer free. Where their original biopsy had shown hopeless cancer, they now had biopsies with no cancer at all!

My own life turned around as I saw hundreds of people go from terminal disease to health. Listening to my students and seeing what they'd done taught me how to be a health teacher. I became a student of my own students and learned from them how to teach health and shared in their joy as they forged a new, healthy life from the seeds of cancer. It was an incredible experience.

How I Was Commanded to Write This Book

In July 1991, Dr. Broeringmeyer passed on. It was a tremendous blow. His wife Mary, who was also a chiropractor, decided to continue his workshops. I gave up workshops myself, not wanting to be in competition with Mary.

I did not continue with my Biohealth Program. I'd been stunned by Richard's death, and I went on to other things.

Then it happened. On December 8, 1995, at University Hospital in Cleveland, I had a biopsy of my prostate gland done. I was diagnosed with advanced prostate cancer.

At University Hospital "advanced" is a nice way of saying "terminal." The biopsy showed that 45 percent of my prostate gland consisted of cancer cells. There was also perineural invasion, meaning that nerves had been invaded by the cancer cells and the cancer had spread outside the prostate gland.

Since the cancer had metastasized (spread) beyond the prostate gland, no treatment was possible. I was given a death sentence. When prostate cancer cannot be treated, the patient is given a medication called lupron. Lupron does not remove or kill the cancer but slows it down by stopping the production of testosterone. It is a chemical castration. I was put on lupron and told I might have a year. No longer.

I immediately went on the Biohealth cancer program outlined in this book. At the end of one year, I was still alive. In fact, I was getting better. Because of this, after 15 months on the lupron, against the strong advice of my urologist, I decided to quit taking it. My urologist said this could be fatal. But my urologist had not seen my Biohealth readings. My own body, through these readings, was telling me I was getting healthier. Cancer cannot grow in a healthy body. So, rather than do what my urologist said to do (which was medically correct), I did what my body told me to do.

At the end of two years my Biohealth readings no longer showed cancer. I asked to have another biopsy of my prostate gland. This was done on November 20, 1997. *It showed no cancer.* Just as had happened to so many people Dr. Richard and I worked with, the cancer had been replaced by healthy cells.

Now I had some questions to answer. Since I could have prevented the cancer why had I not done so? And why did I develop terminal cancer at all? What was my cancer telling me? What was I supposed to do with the information I'd gained?

In a quiet and unexpected moment a few months later, I got my answer. My cancer and my survival was a loud and clear *command* to make the knowledge of biological health and the Biohealth System available to anyone who wants it.

You are holding the results of that command in your hand right now. If you are excited and interested in taking control of your own health and life, it's time to strap on your seat belt, get into this book and prepare to fly!

The Biohealth System is incredible. It provides the keys to total health and a new understanding of your body, an understanding that most of us never knew existed. I should know. It saved me. It returned me to health. And it can do the same thing for you.

How to Get the Most Out of This Book

There are three kinds of chapters in this book. Chapters 1 through 9 are background chapters. Chapters 1 through 5 give an overview of the science and philosophy behind the Biohealth System. Chapters 6 through 8 present the principles of magnetic testing, which is at the heart of the system. Chapter 9 asks an important question you must truthfully answer: Do you have the right attitude and the courage to become totally healthy? It takes both.

Chapters 10 through 13 are the interactive, nuts-and-bolts chapters of the Biohealth System. In chapters 10 through 13, the step-by-step procedures of the Biohealth Program are outlined.

Chapters 14 and 15 offer support information that deals with Biohealth applications for specific diseases and allied health disciplines that increase the effectiveness of the Biohealth Program. Much of the information in chapters 10 through 15 is quite unique. You're not going to find anything like it anywhere else.

Since everyone is an individual with their own special needs and nature, there will be as many approaches to reading this book as there are readers. That said, there are four general ways to approach it.

The first, the traditional way, is to read all chapters in the sequence in which they are presented. Start with Chapter 1 and read straight through to the end of the book.

The second, and this is important to those who may get impatient with background material, is to skip or skim over the background chapters and proceed directly to the interactive material in chapters 10 through 13. This will give the "go-getters" a chance to get right into the mechanics of the Biohealth System. Later, they can go back to the chapters they skipped, keeping in mind that the material on magnetism in chapters 6 through 8 is important.

The third way to use this book is to alternate between background, interactive and support chapters as desired. That way you can package the information to best serve your needs and preferences.

The fourth way is reserved for those with the strongest needs. *If you have a serious health problem and wish to begin the program immediately, go directly to chapters 10 through 13.* With serious diseases time can be critical, and the sooner you begin using the Biohealth System the better. If the problem is cancer, heart disease or pain, Chapter 14 is very important to you.

Whatever your situation, the important thing is to do what you feel is best for YOU. Where medical and science writings on the subjects of health and disease are often obscure and overloaded with medical jargon, we've chosen to take another road here. Biohealth is not difficult to understand or achieve and we're not going to make it more difficult in an effort to add false credibility. My objective is to present the Biohealth Program in simple language anyone can understand and put to immediate use.

The fact is, whichever method you choose to read this book, you'll find that the great truths of Biohealth and energy balancing are revealed naturally and easily, *through a growing understanding of your own body and how it works.*

Very Important for Health Professionals and All Other Readers

This book is an indepth presentation of the Biohealth System. However, it is written as simply as possible and without technical jargon so as to be easily understood by all.

For the health professional it may seem oversimplified. However, in spite of its simplicity, this book gives the health professional everything she/he needs in order to effectively apply the Biohealth System, and then add their knowledge and experience to it.

Very Important for the Patient and Biohealth Student

Many of the people Dr. Richard Broeringmeyer and I saw began by taking our one-day workshop. This is the best possible way to get started in applying the Biohealth program. However, almost all of you reading this book have not had this opportunity.

Even for those who did take our workshop, Dr. Richard and I always recommended working with a Biohealth trained professional where such a person was available. While I believe I touched all the bases in this book, the experience and knowledge of a trained Biohealth professional will add to the knowledge and ability of the reader of this book.

8

Having the Biohealth professional and the student work together has been very successful. Under the guidance of the professional, the student takes readings at her/his home. To achieve the best therapy and teaching, we prefer the student write down his/her findings and interpretation of those findings, and then discuss them with their Biohealth professional.

With this interaction, each time the Biohealth student and the Biohealth professional get together, the student becomes a better student, and the Biohealth professional becomes a better therapist and guide.

What Is the Biohealth Program?

The goal of the Biohealth Program is both removal of disease and achievement of health. The Biohealth Program is not complete until your body is in a state of health and can maintain itself in health. In today's highly technological world of medicine, we are seen as a group of organs and diseases rather than a powerfully self-healing human being. Instead of using our own enormous inner powers of healing and health, we have turned our powers off by giving them to health professionals. The Biohealth Program uses technological medicine in support of the enormous self-healing powers—not in the replacement of them.

The Biohealth Program is built upon the following six precepts:

- A health program must serve the real needs of the people— not the demands of the economic system

- A new relationship must be established between patients and health professionals

- The mutual separation between patients and health professionals must be replaced by solidarity

- The aim of all disease and health programs must be human well-being and immunity to disease

- At the conclusion of the health program your own body must be able to keep itself in a state of health

- The individual must take an active part in the program

I wish you good luck on the wonderful journey that lies ahead of you—a journey into a world of health, knowledge and self-empowerment that most have never even imagined existed.

CHAPTER 1

Five Medical Myths That Make Biohealth a Necessity for You

What is man's privilege, his exceptional achievement? Consciousness and again consciousness, and it is in a passionate imaginative consciousness that our true rewards are won.

—Llewelyn Powys, *Now That The Gods Are Dead*

It is not the point of this chapter to find fault with modern doctors. Many health professionals are doing a great deal to keep people alive and breathing. Most doctors and health professionals live lives of remarkable compassion, care and concern for their patients and the world around them. They do much good and important work. In this chapter we will define "medical myths" as beliefs about achieving health that are incorrect and misleading.

The research being done in health today produces new information and opens new fields almost daily. In this rapidly growing area no single health program is definitive and has all

11

the answers. Some health programs claim they have has all the answers to achieving health. That turns me off because it tells me their prime interest is not the patient.

The Biohealth Program is inclusive. We continually look to research and other health professionals to continually improve our programs, and we try to continually improve other programs.

With the rapid changes occurring, knowing what is best for you can be very confusing, and a wrong decision by you or your doctor can be very harmful. That is where the Biohealth Program shines. It eliminates the confusion and it gives you your correct path. With the testing of the Biohealth Program you test the new information, you test other programs and you test doctors and health professionals so that *before you use them* you determine which are right for you.

A key point of the Biohealth System is that before *you do anything you test and determine if it will do you good, no good, or harm.*

The basic goal of the Biohealth System is never competitive. It is always cooperative and aimed at attaining synergy. In fact, if there is a basic "religion" to the Biohealth System it is synergy. We rely on other health professionals as needed to make our program the best it can be.

There are six generally believed health myths that can make achieving total health very difficult, if not impossible. Why do so many of us believe these myths?

We've all been indoctrinated with these beliefs through TV, newspapers, magazines, the Internet and other forms of mass media from our first moments of consciousness. Unfortunately, some of these beliefs make it almost impossible to understand what health is and how to achieve it. They make it almost impossible to attain true health.

Let's review these six myths and see how they differ from those of the Biohealth System:

1. Your doctor or other health professionals are the only ones who have the knowledge and ability to bring you health. You do not and cannot have this ability.

2. Drugs cure disease.

3. Medicine is based on hard science.

4. You are exactly like everybody else.

5. Today's test is just the same as yesterday's.

6. Your body is monistic. You are only a physical body. When you treat your physical body you are treating your total body.

Belief in these myths will prevent you from understanding and making full use of the Biohealth System. They may help you control some diseases, but you will not achieve total body health with them. As a result, your first step toward health and immunity from disease, is not to learn but to *unlearn* these six myths.

There's an old saying used in the agriculture field that bears repeating here: "Don't plant the tree until you prepare the soil." In this first chapter we'll prepare the Biohealth soil by extracting some rocks and other medical pollutants from it. That completed, we'll be better able to successfully plant a Biohealth "tree" in the chapters to come.

Medical Myth 1: Your doctor or other health professionals are the only ones who have the knowledge and ability to bring you health. You do not and cannot have this ability.

By much of the health profession and the mass media, you are told that to achieve health you must go to a highly trained health professional and do exactly what he or she tells you to do. Most people accept this. They're perfectly content to play a passive role in their own health. "Fix me," they tell their doctor and she or he does. Or tries. Once they walk through the office door they're just patients, after all. They don't want to have any responsibility for getting healthy. "We'll just let the doctor take care of it while I go on with the rest of my life," they think. It's almost as if our lives and the body treated by the doctor are totally separate, independent things.

I run into this attitude all the time. The fact is, many people don't want to take responsibility for their lives today. They're afraid. They feel helpless. Faced with a society and attendant media that emphasize their shortcomings, their "needs" and their inability to satisfy them, they're taught not to rely on themselves. When in doubt, they go to the "experts."

Meanwhile, medicine has become so successful at alleviating symptoms and making us feel "better" that we have actually come to prefer this "virtual health" to real health. Too bad they don't realize that the best expert on their health is the guy looking back at them in the mirror every morning. In the Biohealth System, you will learn something that most doctors and health professionals don't know: *The greatest health expert you can turn to is your own body.*

Still, there's that pesky belief that the doctor is actually omniscient. They know more about your body than your own body does. "If this treatment was any good, my doctor would know about it," we think. After all, doctors are omniscient. They know all, don't they?

Or do they?

Medical Myth 2: *Drugs cure disease.*

Much of modern medicine relies on the use of drugs. Go to a doctor with an illness and you can be pretty sure you'll be leaving his or her office with a prescription. And it will work— at least partly. The drugs will take away the pain. They'll knock down the symptoms. They'll allow you to live a "normal" life.

But do they really cure?

Too often, they don't. The result of modern medicine's reliance on drugs is that we have a lot of people breathing, walking around and even enjoying life while still sick. The drugs eventually become an addiction, needed to survive. Meanwhile, they're merely palliative. Take them away and you're right back where you started.

Drugs fit right in with modern medicine's focus on an invasive approach to health. The perception is that the causes of disease come from outside the body. So do the cures.

Biohealth emphasizes that diseases originate within the body as a result of people creating the internal environment in which diseases exist. Therefore, cure for that disease must be initiated from within the body by creating an internal environment that produces health and is immune to disease.

Research has shown that the inner environment of your body is like soil. Good soil grows healthy plants. Poor soil grows weak and sick plants. The soil inside your body is your bioenergy. The prefix *bio* means life. Energy by definition is the power to activate. Therefore, bioenergy is the energy of life. It is the power within your body that produces life. Your bioenergy is the energy that originally gave you life and now keeps you alive. It is also the power that produces health.

Bioenergy that is balanced grows health. When your bioenergy is out of balance you cannot grow health, and in an environment in which you cannot grow health disease will grow. Likewise, disease cannot grow in the bioenergy in which health grows.

The entire Biohealth System is based on achieving a bioenergy within your body that grows health. At this time this may sound confusing, but in chapters 10 through 13 you will actually do it! *All health begins in a soil of correct bioenergy.* I know of no system other than Biohealth that, step-by-step, has you produce within your body the bioenergy that can grow only health.

Biohealth directly deals with the causes of disease. Medicine is too often centered on symptoms. Its approach is generally to give you a drug that's not a part of your body, or any other living thing for that matter, to treat the disease. The drug then acts on the damaged part of your body in a way to make the disease less damaging. But it doesn't treat the cause of the disease or the

15

malfunctioning tissue. Drugs do not achieve the bioenergy of health.

For instance, suppose you have a gland that normally secretes healthy substance A. Suddenly, it starts producing a substance B that is harmful to the body. Modern medicine's approach is to give you a drug to change the biochemistry of your body so that you can live with substance B. The gland continues to produce B, which is usually very harmful, but the drug lessens the effects of B so it is less destructive. You may be out of danger, you may feel much better, but you've still got the original problem. Your glands are still producing substance B. Without the drugs, you're right back where you started.

In fact, drugs eat into your body's ability to achieve and maintain health. While the drugs may make you feel better, your glands are still producing substance B and not producing substance A, which they were designed to produce. After a time the gland loses its ability to produce substance A. Now, for the rest of your life, you are dependent on the drug that controls substance B.

Instead of palliating harmful B with a drug so it's not as damaging, Biohealth looks at the energy that's causing your gland to malfunction and determine what you need to do so that your gland is again producing the healthy, natural A instead of the B. The aim of Biohealth is to restore proper body function and total health instead of the "vicarious health" produced by drugs.

Biological health is a health from within rather than without. Biological health is health that is produced and maintained by your own body.

Medical Myth 3: Medicine is based on hard science.

The public, and even doctors themselves, believe strongly that medicine and its daily practice are built on the principles of science. But are they really?

The scientific method involves, by definition, six components:

1. Recognition of a problem.

2. Collection of data through observation and experimentation.

3. Using the data to propose a solution.

4. Applying the solution to the problem.

5. Evaluating results of the applied solution.

6. Proving or disproving your evaluation by further observation and experimentation.

Certainly, most medical research begins at point 1. It starts with the recognition of a health problem. After that, however, science is too often sacrificed to statistics, which are quite simply not science. With no individual observation or experimentation, you give a test drug to a group of sick people. Then you wait to see if they get better. If you test 1,000 people with the drug and 900 get better, the results indicate that the drug cures the disease. *Voilà!* It's all statistics. The individual subjects in these studies are, obviously, going to be very different from each other. Statistics rule. Individual characteristics and responses are ignored and people become nothing more than numbers to be crunched. Sometimes quite creatively. In turn, the drugs tested and approved are given to equally nameless, numbered people in the general population.

This isn't science.

With the Biohealth System, anytime the individual uses a test magnet and it tells the individual to do something, it constitutes an experiment. It's scientific. First, we determine if an organ is functioning properly. If there's something wrong (step 1 of the scientific method defined above) we test to get the data needed to see what will bring it to normal for the individual (steps 2 and 3). Then we do what is necessary to bring it to normal and evaluate what has happened to insure that we've achieved the desired result (steps 4 and 5). Finally, we prove our results (step 6). By following these six steps, you've got a procedure that is 100 percent scientific.

Yes, the Biohealth System is 100 percent hard science.

Face it, statistics aren't science. Even given the crutches of control groups, double blind studies and other "bias reducing" agents, these studies remain *statistical and not scientific.* You cannot draw scientific conclusions from statistical data. To properly perform experimentation you must use a person, not a piece of paper. Proof is in people, not numbers.

Medical Myth #4: You are exactly like everybody else.

This is an assumption made in the drug studies discussed above and it's also the basis for much medical treatment. You are supposed to be like everybody else. Because you are just like everybody else, whatever treatment worked for them will work for you. If it doesn't, something is wrong with you. Right?

Nothing could be further from the truth.

Two of the most important books I've ever read were written by respected biochemist Dr. Roger Williams: *Biochemical Individuality* and *The Wonderful World Within You.* Dr. Williams found that if you want to get at the cause of any disease it has to be done on an individual basis. If you're going to focus only on the manifestations of diseases, called symptoms, you can use powerful drugs to treat masses of people. But if your objective is to achieve any individual's total body health, you've got to look at the individual.

The important principle here is that everybody is unique. As such, no two people have the same needs. For proper health, each person requires an individual assessment of their needs.

Nutritionally, Williams would have thought it silly to prescribe the same low-fat diet for everyone. Or a vegetarian regimen. Or a high-fat diet. Or any diet. Everyone has different needs. The diet that brings health to one person, might not work for another.

In *The Wonderful World Within You,* Dr. Williams also emphasized the importance of a person having knowledge of their own body and how it works. Because your body is not like anybody else's, it is essential for you to know your unique nature and what you need to achieve optimum health.

This fits perfectly into the Biohealth System. Biohealth enables you to know your body and learn how it functions best. Apart from what doctors may indicate, your body's needs are unique. The biochemistry and physiology medicine focuses on is not unique, but the biochemistry and bioenergy of your body is.

With Biohealth, there's no guesswork. You're not dependent on anyone else to tell you what your body needs. You're not dealing with statistics or somebody else's body or an idea of what your body should be. You're dealing with reality.

Medical Myth 5: *Today's test is just the same as yesterday's.*

It's very important to realize that all medical tests are static tests. They tell you what's happening in your body at the moment the tests are given, but that is not necessarily a true picture of your health.

Given the stress and conditions under which a person is living, medical tests can show different results under different conditions. They can change from day to day. What is health under one condition may not be health under another.

In the Biohealth Program, you use a test magnet to test your level of health. You test your health under various conditions and at various times. Nothing and no one can give you the information you can get from your own testing. The information you get when you test is unique to you.

Another great thing about the test magnet is that you test yourself. You don't have to wait for a doctor to perform a test. You don't have to wait to get the results of the test. You can monitor your health as often as you desire.

With the Biohealth System you can determine both how your body is functioning and what it needs to move to a higher level of health. That's one of the reasons the test magnet is such a marvelous instrument. The same magnet you use in testing your body's health is also used to determine your body's nutritional and other needs. There's no guessing. By using the test magnet you ask your body what it needs and it tells you exactly what it needs to produce health.

Unlike medical tests that must be performed by people with a couple degrees and years of training, anybody can learn to use the test magnet. Its principles can be mastered quite quickly as you'll see later in this book. All you need is the will to try something new and a commitment to take responsibility for your own life and health.

Medical Myth 6: *Your body is monistic. You are only a physical body. When you treat your physical body you are treating your total body.*

Modern medicine sees only a part of the picture. Modern medicine limits itself to the world of our five senses. It views people only in terms of the physical body. If it can't be seen, heard, weighed, touched, tasted, smelled or otherwise measured it doesn't exist. Like most people, doctors assume that the human body we live in consists entirely of material elements. We are only solid matter. But is that really accurate?

Physics and research have shown us that our bodies are primarily energy and only a small part of it is solid matter. The nonmaterial part of our body, our bioenergy, is very much greater than the material part, and that's a fact.

Medical science has said that the part of the body which is nonmaterial, our bioenergy, is of little real significance. It continues to view the human body as a collection of material parts. And when problems occur, they do so in a specific material part of our body. So we have a liver problem or a pancreas problem and so forth. This creates a body that has no nonmaterial part— and no bioenergy.

Monism by definition is a view that a complete entity is basically one. Modern medicine and health therapy have converted our body into a monism that is entirely solid matter and has eliminated the nonmaterial bioenergy that science has proven to be by far the largest part of our bodies.

20

Biohealth has overcome this monistic view of our body by showing how the material and nonmaterial parts of our bodies exist as one complete, functioning system. Biohealth sees the body as one organ consisting of both material and nonmaterial elements. Therefore, rather than concentrating only on the material part of our body, Biohealth looks at our entire body, both material and bioenergy.

Rather than designing a separate program for every material part of our body, Biohealth designs health programs for the entire body. Bioenergy and material. Or more accurately, in the Biohealth System, *you* design health programs for *your* entire body. In the patient-centered approach, which dominates traditional medicine, we think the answer to health lies outside of us. In the Biohealth System, you directly communicate with both your bioenergy self and your physical self. You come to understand that the only thing that can really heal your body is your own body and you are ultimately responsible for creating an environment in your body in which optimal health exists. As such, you then begin to take control of your body, health and life.

This means using your own experience and intelligence to seek and find real answers, not just temporary solutions or a drug crutch. It means taking the responsibility for your own health and moving to a higher level of living and knowing.

If Biohealth sounds exciting to you, please read on.

CHAPTER 2

The Biohealth System–Adventures in the Body Electric

To have been born, that is a chance that outweighs all; and the wise man recognizes a sacred obligation to each brief moment.

—Llewelyn Powys, *Now That The Gods Are Dead*

Biological health, or *Biohealth*, is all about energy.

Like most people, doctors assume that the world we live in, including your body and your health, consists entirely of the material elements. Modern medicine limits itself to the world of our five senses. It views man only in terms of the physical world and physical body. If it can't be seen, heard, weighed, touched, tasted, smelled or otherwise measured it doesn't exist. But is that really accurate?

Quantum physics and astrophysics have given us the answer. They have shown us that our world is made up of small particles called *quarks*. There are two kinds of quarks. One kind is material and makes up the matter, the solid stuff, that our world is made out of. These are the quarks we "see" with our five physical senses.

The other kind of quark is nonmaterial and it makes up the energy that fills our universe. Since none of our five senses is aware of the nonmaterial quarks, we call them empty space. Actually, that "empty" space is the most filled space in the universe. It is filled with energy.

How much of the universe we live in is material (solid matter), and how much is nonmaterial (energy)? Science has shown that by far the nonmaterial quarks make up most of our universe. In fact, *out of every 100 million quarks that make up our universe, only one is matter.* The other 99,999,999 particles are *energy.* Therefore, only 0.0001 percent of our universe is material. The other 99.9999 percent is nonmaterial. When we use our five physical senses we are in contact with only our material world, meaning we are in contact with 0.0001 percent of the universe in which we live.

(For those wanting a more scientific explanation of this, I recommend an exciting book by Nobel Prize winner Leon Lederman, *The God Particle.* See page 286 of this book.)

Our human body is made up of over 100 trillion cells. Each cell is composed similar to our universe. In fact, each cell can be seen as a tiny living universe. There is a little bit of matter in the nucleus of the cell, and the huge majority of the cell is bioenergy. Just as our universe is almost entirely energy, every cell in our body is almost entirely energy.

Since the energy that fills our cells produces our life and health, we call it bioenergy, the energy of life. When your bioenergy is correct and in balance, neither too much nor too little, nor too strong nor too weak, you have health. Possessing this balance is the basis of health. Your body is composed of over 100 trillion cells. Every second each of these cells performs over a million chemical reactions. In addition to its own correct chemical reactions, each cell must also keep its chemical reactions in harmony with the chemical reactions of all the other 100 trillion cells in your body.

Obviously, the complexity of managing all of these chemical reactions simultaneously is well beyond what any person or any human technology can now do. *Only your own body has the knowledge and technological capability to manage all this and keep your body in health.*

The Biohealth System balances the bioenergy in your body. This is the beginning of all health. When your bioenergy is balanced, it produces correct body function. With correct body function, the biochemistry of your material body is correct and you have health.

When bioenergy is out of balance it cannot produce correct body function. Instead, it produces malfunction. With malfunction, the biochemistry and physiology of your material body is incorrect and disease results. Disease cannot exist in a body whose bioenergy is balanced. Health cannot exist in a body that is out of balance. Therefore, balanced bioenergy is the soil that grows healthy bodies, and unbalanced bioenergy is the soil that grows diseased bodies.

In the Biohealth System the first thing you will learn to do is to balance your bioenergy. Then you will learn how to give your body what it needs so that your own body will balance your bioenergy. When your own body, without outside help, produces balanced bioenergy you have biological health, or Biohealth. Balanced bioenergy is the basis of all health. Since health and disease cannot exist in the same body at the same time, balanced bioenergy both produces health and makes you immune to disease. As long as your body maintains balanced bioenergy, you have high immunity to disease.

What Does the Biohealth System Do That Other Systems Don't Do?

First, it is a step-by-step health program in which you do the steps that bring you health. You do not pass responsibility for your health and life over to any other person. You are not at the mercy of any health professional or medical test. You are not in the position of blindly trusting somebody else to make health decisions for you. You do the program yourself and rely on the greatest health expert of all—your own body—to make your health decisions for you.

Second, the Biohealth Program concentrates not on your physical body but on your inner bioenergy body. Modern medicine pays no attention to your bioenergy. It uses drugs to offset any malfunctions present. Since drugs don't really correct the malfunctions present you often continue to take drugs indefinitely. Since, without bioenergy balance, the drugs are necessary for your body to function well, you are addicted to the drugs.

As long as you take the drugs, the symptoms and the effects of the malfunctions may be masked and controlled, but as soon as you go off the drugs, symptoms return and you can find yourself as sick as you were. Therefore, your need for drugs sends an important message to you. It tells you that, though you may feel and function much better, your bioenergy is still out of balance and your physical body is not functioning properly. In essence, you're still sick.

Modern medicine and most health programs aim at treating symptoms. They treat the immediate malfunctions of your material body. Biohealth aims at restoring the bioenergy imbalances that cause your malfunctions and produce disease. When you have Biohealth, or balanced bioenergy, you have health and high immunity to disease. You're not treating symptoms, you're treating the cause of disease and insuring it won't occur again.

This brings us to the third thing that Biohealth does that other systems do not. With Biohealth, you are in direct contact with and you interact with your own bioenergy body. You determine where your bioenergy is out of balance. You then determine what your body needs for it to restore bioenergy balance and health.

Once restored, *the Biohealth System has you prove you have attained biological health.* No other system I know of has a method of proving that your body itself is producing health. In the final step of the Biohealth Program, you set up a program that will keep your body in bioenergy balance and in health until the day you die.

Starting with Chapter 10, as you go through this book you will be given instructions for completing each of these steps. The goal of the Biohealth System is not to make health an occasional condition occurring in between illnesses. It is to create a healthy body and keep it that way.

The Body Electric

As discussed previously, modern medicine focuses on the material aspects of how the body works—namely its biochemistry and physiology. The nonmaterial part of the body—your bioenergy—is ignored.

The Biohealth System does not bypass or ignore the biochemistry and physiology of your material body. But it treats it realistically. The biochemical changes and physiological malfunctions of your material body that produce disease are caused by imbalances in the bioenergy system of the body. Every harmful biochemical and physiologic change is preceded by a harmful change in bioenergy. It is the imbalances of the body's bioenergy that causes the harmful biochemistry and physiology that produce disease.

Attending to only the material part of the body—its biochemistry and physiology—is the reason why illness becomes chronic. Treating only the pathological biochemistry and paying no attention to the bioenergy that caused the pathological biochemistry creates a body that cannot restore a health producing biochemistry.

Many of the drugs prescribed by modern medicine are substitutes for correct function. People become addicted to them because they don't really correct the cause of the pathological

27

biochemistry. If they go off the drugs, the harmful biochemistry returns to produce disease. Biohealth aims to return the body to proper function instead of substituting a drug for that function.

While medicine may not recognize this fact, the truth is that the living human body runs on electricity. Research described in many books, most recently by Dr. Robert Becker (in his book *The Body Electric—Electromagnetism and the Foundation of Life*), confirms this fact. The electric current in our body doesn't directly control physiology but it joins with its magnetic field to create a bioelectromagnetic field that *does* control your physiology, chemistry, biology and other bodily functions. In fact, your body is controlled by the magnetic field that accompanies its electric current. When you measure your body's magnetic field you are actually measuring its bioelectromagnetic field.

These biomagnetic fields in your body comprise your bioenergy. Indeed, your human body was given life by and is now kept living by these biomagnetic fields. They permeate the entire body. If they are of proper strength and balanced, they produce the biochemistry of health. If not, they produce the biochemistry of disease.

The Biohealth Program gives the body what it needs to produce balanced bioenergy. Like the healthy soil, once bioenergy is in proper strength and balance, it produces health producing biochemistry and physiology.

Essence

Essence by definition is the basic or necessary constituent of a thing; anything's intrinsic nature, as contrasted with that which is accidental, ephemeral or superficial.

Our body is almost entirely made up of bioenergy, and the bioenergy that makes up our body is the bioenergy that created us, gave us life and now keeps us alive and healthy. Since our bioenergy is the basic constituent of our living body, by definition it is our essence.

Every person's essence is unique. Your essence is not just bioenergy, it is the specific bioenergy that created you and you alone. Like fingerprints and handwriting, no two essences are the same. From creation throughout life you are different from every other person on earth. And the reason every person is different from every other person is that no two of us have the same essence. This leads to a key point—*since no two people have exactly the same essence, no two people have the exact same requirements for biological health.*

The health and disease profession does not look at your essence. It looks at your physical body as a chemical machine like anyone else's. Whatever treatment another person receives for illness is generally assumed to work for you as well.

In the Biohealth System you work with your essence, your absolutely and totally unique inner self. Tuning into your essence is reaching into the highest power available in our universe. When you contact your essence, you are contacting the bioenergy that created your life and body.

Disease can be viewed as a command from your essence, or your creator, to correct the imbalances you have produced in your bioenergy. It's also a sure sign that you haven't been communicating and interacting with your essence to ensure proper function. Only by deciding to use the Biohealth System to develop your ability to communicate and to interact with your essence will you come to live your fullest and healthiest possible life. Indeed, making that decision is one of the most important steps you will take in your life.

Your essence is your inner point of power. Your physical body is an expression of your essence. In most medical treatment today the sick person is disempowered and must depend on health professionals.

Biohealth demands the exact opposite approach. With the Biohealth System you turn to your essence, your huge world of inner power, for guidance. When you use your inner power, the power of your essence, you are empowered. Your physical body is that which you see. Your bioenergy body, your essence, is that which you are!

Self-healing is the basis of all healing. Your essence provides you an invisible, ever-renewing, ever-growing source of inner power that produces self-healing. From your essence you draw the information and power needed to take control of the functioning and overall health of your body.

Your body is an incredible miracle. Compare it to a giant symphony orchestra. Every one of those 100 trillion cells that make up your body—every organ, gland, system, every body part—must function properly and be in perfect harmony to produce a healthy body. The conductor of this fantastic symphony, the conductor that keeps it working perfectly and in perfect harmony, is your personal essence.

Because you are unique, your road to health is also unique. The Biohealth System will help you discover this road. Your destiny is in your own hands. Biohealth requires that you *wake up to your inner power and grasp the reins of control*, so you may walk your road to a lifetime of health.

The Biohealth System is much more than a health program. It's a road map to your inner self. A guide to a boundless source of knowledge and strength. A window not only to your own body but to your own origins and identity. Only by seeking out your essence will you achieve full health and reach your highest levels of Biohealth.

Biohealth Can Be Learned By Almost Anyone

The methods and technology of the Biohealth System are simple and easy to use. I've tried to apply the principle of "Occam's razor" to everything in this book. "Occam's razor" states that, all things being equal, the simplest explanation to a phenomenon is the most useful and accurate. All unnecessary explanations and material are thus cut away, leaving us with only the essential.

One of the big reasons why the Biohealth System is so easy to use and understated is the fact that it concentrates on health instead of disease. The Biohealth practitioner knows that health and disease are mutually exclusive. When you have health, you have a body in which disease cannot exist. When you have disease, you have a body in which health cannot exist. Biohealth gives you a reliable, achievable step-by-step program for creating an environment that will produce health in your body.

The Three-Phase Biohealth Program

When you get to chapters 10 through 12 of this book you will be taken through the seven steps of the Biohealth System. Right now, to give you a preview of what you will be doing in chapter 10, I am going to divide the seven steps into three phases.

Whereas much of modern medicine cannot fuse with our bioenergy or "life energy" self, the Biohealth System revolves around an intimate relationship with it. By the time you finish this book you will have the knowledge and ability to make full use of that relationship to *produce and maintain your own health.*

Here is a brief summary of the Biohealth System:

Phase I—Checking How You Are Functioning

The first question you answer in the Biohealth System is, "How is my body now functioning? In chapters 10 and 11 of this book we'll show you, step-by-step, how to determine the areas in your body where bioenergy is unbalanced. You'll learn both how to properly use a test magnet, which is Biohealth's "window to the world within you". You will be given body identification markers on the surface of your body that tell you exactly where to make your bioenergy readings. Once you do this, you move into phase II.

Phase II—Restoring Proper Function and Proving It!

The Biohealth System provides a set of instructions for returning any organ or body part not functioning properly to health.

First, you restore bioenergy balance to areas out of balance. A unique feature of the Biohealth System is that, by using the window provided to you by your test magnet, you can see how effective any nutritional changes and any other treatments will be *before* you use them. This allows you to choose, with precise accuracy, the right program for balancing the bioenergy of an organ and returning normal function to the organ that is malfunctioning.

After restoring bioenergy balance, you must make sure that your own body can produce that balanced energy. In the Biohealth Program this is called "proving." When your body, without outside help, keeps itself in bioenergy balance, you know it is both healthy and immune to future disease. The last step in phase II is to prove, not guess, that your body is now balancing its bioenergy.

You'll also know that you're ready for phase III.

Phase III—Maintaining Correct Function

The purpose of the Biohealth System is not only to restore correct function but to keep it that way. In phase III you monitor your bioenergy balance, and therefore your health, for the rest of your life. You become older but successfully avoid those diseases and difficulties many people call "aging."

Advantages of the Biohealth System

We've already discussed many advantages of the Biohealth System. It is designed for you alone. It gives you control of your own life and health. It can be used by almost everyone. It changes as often as your needs or the stress in your life changes. It's inexpensive. Natural. Painless. Convenient.

There are additional advantages. The first is that the Biohealth System is accurate and noninvasive. You already know there are no drugs or needles or surgical procedures associated with Biohealth. You should also know that, unlike X-rays, which are invasive and at best give you a two-dimensional picture of a three-dimensional organ, the Biohealth System actually allows you to "see" how each part of your body is working. Knowing this, you can continually correct energy imbalances and keep your entire body functioning correctly over the course of time.

When a Biohealth correcting magnet is placed over an organ the magnetic energy goes directly to that organ. *Nothing stops magnetic energy.* It goes through anything. The only thing that will stop magnetic energy is distance, which doesn't become a factor in the Biohealth System.

Another advantage of the Biohealth System comes from its focus on self-empowerment. Because you are in control of your own life and health, *you do not need to grieve over illness.* Illness is a wake-up call to tell you to get to work. With the Biohealth System you listen to the message provided by your illness and give your body what it is asking for so it can produce the balanced bioenergy and health it is designed to. You don't wait around sulking, feeling sorry for yourself and helpless. You take control.

The Biohealth System allows you to pursue "internal health". As defined by the Biohealth System, health is internal not external. With external health, the recipient (the patient) accepts what is offered because the provider knows best. This approach doesn't promote understanding or knowledge. It is a subtractive process, where personal power and the recipient's knowledge are diminished, and their dependency is increased.

Biohealth is a growth process where the understanding and the power and knowledge of the recipient are increased. The only way to fuse our bioenergy nonmaterial essence with our biochemistry material self is to directly communicate with our essence and achieve "internal" health. "Internal" health is the balancing of your bioenergy and is the beginning of true health.

Your bioenergy self controls the biochemistry of your material body, and by producing correct biochemistry produces health. Internal health is true health. And only the Biohealth System puts you in touch with your internal health channels.

What About Aging?

A major issue for people today is aging. People are living longer and want to stay healthy longer. Yet we live in a consumer-oriented, media-driven society where youth is prized and age often despised. It's also assumed that age goes hand-in-hand with frailty and disease. From our youth, we learn to fear it and attach to it so many negatives.

Certainly, there are changes that occur as we grow older. In youth, the body has tremendous abilities to maintain its energy balances through almost bottomless organic reserves. Your body is at its strongest between the ages of 25 and 30. From then on, each year your body metabolism slows down and your organ reserves diminish. Your ability to automatically maintain balanced energy fields lessens. Many people come to believe that, as they grow older, they have no choice but to be besieged by disease and ultimately forced to live life on drugs to compensate for poor body function.

But what we've come to call "aging" is not really aging at all but a collection of diseases and health problems that we are more prone to as our bodies get older. And while the probability of experiencing these diseases increases with age, we do not have to give in to disease. Indeed, by using the Biohealth System we can keep our bioenergy fields in balance.

The mission of the Biohealth System is to have you live your entire life span with the "youngest" body possible, free of the diseases of "old age." When you die, and that is an inevitable part of our life's journey, we want you to have lived your life with your youngest and happiest body possible.

Don't let anybody tell you differently. There is such a thing as "growing older without aging" and with the Biohealth System you achieve it.

What About Genetics?

Throughout medical history two unquestioned rules have served as the basis for the science of genetics.

The first rule is that we are who we are because of the genes we got from our parents. These genes determine personality, physique, how healthy we will be and how long we will live. They also control the production and day-to-day function of all cells in our body.

The second rule is that nothing can change these genes. It's all our parents' fault. Like the doctors we choose to cure us, our parents control our lives and health through their genetic legacy. This is very convenient. Between the doctors and our parents, we don't have to take responsibility for anything. It's never our fault.

And what a tremendous array of genes we have to blame. We've got heart attack genes, cancer genes, diabetes genes, height genes, weight genes, longevity genes, Levi's jeans (oops, I guess we can't blame anybody for those). And woe to us if we've been given a bad set of genes. Genetic law says we can't change those bad genes into good ones. We're doomed.

Thank goodness for medicine! If we get stuck with bad genes, at least they'll be there to heroically intervene and keep us out of pain and on our feet.

But do genes really constitute our destiny?

As we become older our genes obviously change. We are an expression of our genetic function. When we are 25 years old we have the genes of a 25-year-old. When we are 70, we have the genes of a 70-year-old. We cannot reach age 70 and turn our genes magically back to 30-year-old genes. In time, our genes go only in one direction and that is toward becoming older.

Recent research shows that specific changes in our genes are related to specific diseases. However, it also shows that the *genes themselves do not produce disease*. Our genes produce a predisposition toward disease, but they aren't a death sentence. Disease is not expressed until the person is plunged into a harmful environment. Without the harmful environment the disease does not occur. Genes may set the stage, but it is the harmful environment that produces the disease.

35

The Rules Are Wrong

Here's where that first rule of genetics starts to lose its credibility. Our parents don't genetically determine exactly who we become. Indeed, the fact that as we grow older our genes change in a way that makes us more susceptible to disease disproves the rule of genetic determinism. *Since our genes continually change as we get older, they are obviously plastic. They do change!*

Not only that, it's apparent from research that many of the genetic changes that occur as we get older are modifiable. By knowing what to do, we can bring about changes in our genetic function. *The old first rule of genetics that says we can't change our genetic function is wrong!*

The magnetic research of Albert Roy Davis, which will be discussed later, and the success of the Biohealth System prove that when we restore balanced bioenergy, older genes can function as younger genes.

Which brings us to the second rule of genetics that says genetics are irreversible. Once a cell matures and ages and becomes more differentiated and complicated, it can never revert back to being a simpler cell. Or so said the genetics field.

But the cloning of Dolly the sheep in Scotland in 1997 showed us that our genes aren't locked in stone. They can be changed. In the cloning of Dolly, differentiated cells were reversed into more primitive cells making the cloning possible. It was also discovered that, while some kinds of genes cannot be modified very much, others can be substantially changed. And changed in many directions.

Genes send messages to our body that control how our body functions, how we age, how susceptible to disease we are, how long we'll live and countless other things. Dolly showed us we can change those messages. If we do not like the way things are going, we can often replace those messages we don't like with ones we do.

This is tremendously empowering knowledge. Once we go beyond the discredited and obsolete rules of genetic determinism and irreversibility we open up a whole new concept of health. We can change the messages our genes send.

Another recent health breakthrough was the discovery that nutrition significantly modifies genetic function. This was considered a remarkable breakthrough for scientists but many nonscientists have known about it for some time. In fact, we've all known for decades that nutrition, among several other lifestyle factors, can affect genetic function. We all know that if you eat too much you get fat and a diet full of refined carbohydrates increases your chance of disease markedly. Environmental stress provides an obvious opportunity for the development of disease. Smoking increases the chance of heart disease and alcohol increases the characteristics of aging. I could go on and on.

What's important to realize here is that many things—our diets, our response to stress, our environment, our beliefs, our exercise patterns and so forth—all affect genetic function. *And they can all be modified.*

Even more important is the knowledge that, *with the Biohealth System, we can directly speak to our genes and tell them how we want them to function.* Your bioenergy fields help determine gene function. An imbalanced field produces defective gene function. But by balancing bioenergy, we improve and restore gene function.

Chronological and Biological Age

What is the difference between chronological and biological age. Chronological age is a matter of arithmetic. It simply measures how many years you've lived. Biological age can be very different. It measures how old or young your body is functioning.

A man of age 50 may possess a biological age of 70. Likewise, a man of 70 may possess a biological age of 50. Chronological age measures the number of years you've lived. Biological age measures the quality of life you are now living. It's much more important than your chronological age.

Here's where genetics come in again. They are important to biological age but they can be changed. According to recent research in functional medicine, 75 percent of your health after age 50 can be modified. That is to say that 75 percent of the genetic function that produces disease or health in our "senior citizens" *can be changed.* You are not locked into health problems by unchangeable genes. You can modify the health patterns your genes produce. You can keep them at their youngest and healthiest.

The truth is that at any chronological age, we are capable of producing a younger biological age. We can alter genetic function away from susceptibility to disease and toward health. If you don't like disease, misery, fatigue, pain and the other problems we've long believed come with aging, you have the capability of determining what is causing your genes to produce these problems and making changes so that your genetic function will produce health, vitality and the life you desire.

How do you do this? When you use the Biohealth System you change your genetic function. That's what you will do as you progress in this book. In fact, in Chapter 10 you'll begin to speak directly to your genes! As you work through Chapter 10 you will directly improve your genetic function! Sound exciting?

Guidance

Trained health professionals have information and experience you do not. They can be of great help to you. But it's very important you find the right professional. Above all, you want a health professional who won't make you into a passive participant. You want a health professional who knows that self-healing is possible. You want a health professional who will look at your total person—not just an illness—and be a guide not a dictator. When you've got someone who feels that educating and empowering you is a critical part of the service she or he is performing for you, you're on the right track.

One of the great things about the Biohealth System is that it gives you a way to test what your health professional is doing for you. Through Biohealth testing you'll know if what's being done for you is helping, harming or doing nothing at all. The Biohealth System not only tests your own health. It also tests your health care professional. The number one requirement for any health professional is that he or she pass the Biohealth test and *prove* that whatever treatment they've offered is helping you.

There are also many classes, workshops and books that can provide information and guidance. They can be very helpful but, again, they should only be used when your testing *proves* that what they are telling you to do improves your health. *There is no more important key to health than the Biohealth testing you will do.* The bottom line is always: Does whatever you're doing restore bioenergy balance.

It is essential not to believe any health professional, class, method or book (including this one) until *you prove it through Biohealth testing!*

Finding and Using Your Inner Teacher

While it's certainly true that health professionals and writers can aid you in your pursuit of health, it's important to realize and remember there's no way they'll ever be able to teach you anything close to what your own body can. Your "inner teacher" is the greatest teacher of all.

Only your own body can tell you where you have balanced energy and where you do not. Only your own body can tell you what it needs to produce balanced energy. Your objective in the Biohealth System is to tune into the greatest miracle on earth—your own body—and listen and learn from its limitless knowledge.

When you interact with your essence and begin to look through the Biohealth window into your own bioenergy fields, a whole new world will open up. You will develop a tremendous admiration for your own body. You will learn to more fully ex-

39

perience it. You will learn that it is your best teacher and a great friend.

Today, because of our reliance on experts, we have lost contact with our bodies. The Biohealth System restores contact between you and your body and rebuilds your relationship with it. Ultimately, the Biohealth System puts you in a state of continual conversation with your own body. Health professionals, books and other methods can be important but none can ever take the place of the most important and essential guide to your own bioenergy, your inner self. The lessons taught you by your great "inner teacher" are the most important the Biohealth System has to offer.

Breaking Free—Clearing the Hurdle Between You and Your Inner Teacher

Allow me to illustrate the situation faced by most people today. Take, for example, a group of common houseflies. A jar is filled with the flies and a lid put on the jar. The flies are regularly fed and they remain healthy but the lid prevents them from flying out of the jar.

Later, the lid is removed from the jar but only a few flies choose to fly out. The physical obstruction to their flying from the jar, the lid, has been removed but by now the lid has become a mental obstruction as well. Many times in life, these mental obstructions are just as imposing as the physical variety.

The first step in achieving balanced bioenergy and functional health is to break through the mental obstructions that tell you you cannot interact with your body to produce health. Health professionals and other people who tell you you can't aren't necessarily lying to you. They're being honest. They believe what they say. Since they can't interact with their own bodies to produce health, they assume nobody else can.

But don't believe them. For that matter, don't believe me. All you need to do is break through that mental obstruction provided by others and your own habits and prejudices and try the Biohealth System. You will know they are wrong only when *you* prove it to yourself.

Consider the caterpillar. It lives a very restricted life on a single green leaf. That leaf is its whole world. As the caterpillar matures, a wonderful thing happens. It spins a cocoon. Gradually, the crawling caterpillar disappears until one day a beautiful, glorious, graceful butterfly emerges from the cocoon in its place— endowed with wings. Now, instead of living a life restricted to the leaf, the butterfly soars above the trees—liberated, unrestricted, free to become the wonderful thing it was created and intended to be.

We all start out as that caterpillar. When we learn to use our body as a teacher, it becomes a cocoon. As we learn more and achieve balanced bioenergy and functional health, the caterpillar disappears. Only then do we emerge from the cocoon ready to become the full, healthy human being we were created and intended to be.

In summary then, our physical human body is made of the materials of the earth, but our living human body is from life energy. Every human body is kept alive and healthy by this life energy, which we call bioenergy and/or essence. One who searches for health entirely outside of the human body, and goes no further into the human body than its material outer shell, gets lost.

CHAPTER 3

The Universe You Live In— What Is It? Why Is It? Where Is It Now? Where Is It Going?

To open delicately contrived eyelids on this earth, on this fifth-smallest of the planets, which like a flock of frightened birds keeps sailing around the sun, is surely a chance beyond all chances.

—Llewelyn Powys, *Skin for Skin*

You are your essence. You are the unique life energy that created you. A disease is a command from your essence, your bioenergy and your creator to correct the imbalances you have produced in your bioenergy. Disease and illness tell you you are not communicating and interacting with your essence.

To learn the Biohealth System and communicate more successfully with your essence, it is important to get a larger understanding of the creative energy that comprises your essence. We can do this by gaining a greater knowledge of the creative energy of the universe from which your creative energy came.

What is our universe? How was it created? Where is it going? Your answers to these questions will give you a foundation for understanding how the universe works and how this applies to the Biohealth System.

Since your own energy is just a smaller version of the energy that runs the universe, understanding more about the big picture that is the universe will give insight into the mini-universe within each of us. That's what we'll try to provide in this chapter.

What Is Our Universe?

Science, philosophy and religion all agree that much exists beyond what we can comprehend with our five basic human senses. The material world is the only world available to these senses but that world is only a very tiny part of the universe. The large majority of our universe is energy in the form of electromagnetic radiation.

Since our five senses aren't aware of this energy, we call the space it dwells in "empty space," but it is far from that. In fact, that empty space in which electromagnetic radiation exists may be the most "filled" space in our universe.

Research has shown us that the electromagnetic radiation that fills up our universe is somehow tied to information. In 1984, Dr. Francis Schmitt of the Massachusetts Institute of Technology introduced a term for this information. He called it *information substance* (IS).

There are different explanations for the nature of this information. Schmitt's explanation was that electromagnetic radiation is a *carrier* of information and that this information produces intelligence.

Dr. Tom Stonier, a physicist from England, saw a different explanation of electromagnetic radiation. In his book *Informa-*

tion and the Internal Structure of the Universe, Dr. Stonier states that the electromagnetic energy in our universe does not carry information. He believes it is *made up of information*. This universal information is the energy that created the universe (and us, for that matter) and makes up most of our universe.

Whichever theory of IS you choose to believe, the conclusions are basically the same. The energy that fills our universe provides it with universal information and universal intelligence. In fact, *we live in a sea of universal intelligence*. We were created from that sea of universal intelligence and are kept alive and functioning by it.

Our essence is derived from the IS of the electromagnetic energy of our universe. A major objective of Biohealth is to tune into the IS in that small drop of universal energy that is our essence and use it to promote health and growth.

As fish live in a sea of water, so do we live in a sea of IS. Fish require water to live. We require information and intelligence to become the wonderful thing we were created and intended to be. When we listen to our essence and the body it created, we are in tune with the IS that makes up our sea of universal intelligence.

The Intelligence You Have Available to You Is Infinite

The energy that fills the "empty" space of our universe is in the physical form of electromagnetic radiation. We can verify the existence of this energy because it occurs in waves and waves have lengths (called *frequencies)* and heights (called *amplitude)* that can be measured. From the very shortest electromagnetic waves to the very longest, there is one continuous series of waves. This series of waves is called the *electromagnetic spectrum* and the number of waves within it is infinite.

All these waves travel at an identical speed—the speed of light—which is 186,000 miles per second. But that's where the resemblance ends. Each one of these waves is unique because each has its own frequency, amplitude and form. Therefore, each wave carries a unique intelligence. With each wave carrying a unique intelligence and an infinite number of waves in existence, the intelligence you have available to you is also going to be infinite or as close to the principle of "infinite" as the universe will allow.

There is, then, no limit to the amount of information and growth available to us from our universe.

How Did Our Universe Begin

The Big Bang Theory still offers the best and most accepted conception of the origin of our universe. At the center of this theory is the belief that the universe began with a big explosion called the Big Bang.

Tom Stonier has theorized that, at the time of the Big Bang, the universe was composed almost entirely of disorder and chaos. There was no life, or even matter as we know it, in existence. Nor was there any "information" as we defined it above. But right after the Big Bang event, information began to enter the universe to replace all the disorder. As this occurred about 15 billion years ago, the forces of "nature" began to appear. As more information came into the universe, it was able to create matter.

About 4.7 billion years ago there was sufficient information in our universe to create the earth. Four billion years ago that information reached the level where self-organizing molecules were created. Three billion years ago the first "life" was created in the form of primitive bacteria and tiny blue-green algae. As electromagnetic waves provided more information, more complex life evolved. The earth entered a more creative stage. In the beginning, after the Big Bang, original information entered the universe slowly. It took 10.3 billion years for the earth to be created.

But as more information entered the universe, the speed at which it entered also increased greatly. The first animals and precursors to man appeared and evolved very quickly in contrast to the development of the earth itself. And the speed at which information has entered the universe since then has continued to increase dramatically.

If you have any doubt of this, consider the last 100 years of mankind's history. The Wright Brothers flew the first airplane in 1904. By mid-century we were flying jet airplanes. As the century progressed we went to the moon. Now we have a space station, a shuttle to get there and back, pictures from the Mars landscape and computers that defy imagination to help us explore whatever we want to explore. Before all this we were riding horses and doing arithmetic in paper notebooks.

All this tells us that our universe is not a static thing. It is continually evolving, rapidly growing and creating itself and, as the universe grows older, the information available per unit time rapidly increases. Thus, our universe is evolving more and more rapidly to higher levels of information.

As this occurs, the universe becomes capable of bringing itself into higher and higher levels of intelligence. And the higher the level of intelligence in the universe, the higher the level of intelligence mankind has available for its use. Who knows what this will all lead to in the twenty-first century?

Why Are We Here?

Dr. Stonier's theory leads us to a conception of the universe as an entity created to continually evolve to higher levels of information and intelligence. The universe is not a static thing that was fully created at its origin. It is continually evolving into more. If the purpose of the universe that created us is to continually evolve to higher levels of intelligence, what does that tell you about the purpose of our lives?

Indeed, we tend to grow in much the same way as the universe does. When a child is first born, he or she is not much more evolved than the universe was right after the Big Bang.

47

The child can't write books or use a computer. The child can't fly an airplane. The child can't do much more than lie in a crib.

But as the child receives more information, he or she begins to develop physically and mentally. By adulthood, a person can do all the things mentioned above and many more. Mentally, the only boundaries restricting him or her come from the ability to access and process the universal information and intelligence available. The Biohealth System seeks to unlock that universal intelligence through communication with your essence, which created your human body, and is your window into the universe your essence came from.

And so, like the universe, we continue to achieve higher and higher levels of being. In recent years, the rate of our evolution has dramatically increased. Just as our universe is evolving at a faster and faster pace, we are evolving at a faster and faster rate.

Indeed, the universe has been around for 16 billion years. We've only been around for 2.5 million and look how far we've come. Can there be any doubt we're here to continue to evolve and achieve the highest form of intelligence and existence we can?

The Power of the Atom

Our daily world is made up of seemingly solid matter. We sit in a solid chair that holds us up. We stub our toes on the very same solid chair. We fly in a very solid airplane. We thump our very solid chests. But how solid is our solid world?

The solid matter of our world is made up of atoms. Studies of the composition of atoms show that the amount of matter and energy in the atom is similar to the amount of matter and energy in our universe. Virtually all the matter of the atom is in the nucleus or center of the atom. The size of the nucleus for most atoms is 0.00001 of its total. Thus, each atom is a very large amount of energy combined with a little bit of matter.

This is in perfect harmony with Biohealth's concept of the human body. Since all of us are made up of atoms and atoms consist of a great deal of energy and very little matter, so we are made up of a huge amount of electromagnetic energy and a little bit of matter. But if we have so little matter in us, what makes us solid? What makes the chair we sit in solid? Or the car we drive? Or the paper of this book?

It isn't the matter itself. What makes them solid is electrical energy. These things are all solidly bound together by electricity. This shouldn't be surprising. If you have any doubt about how much energy is contained in the tiny atoms that make up our material world, ask anyone who was in the city of Hiroshima, Japan, at 8:16 A.M. on August 6, 1945. At that moment an atom bomb—a bomb that released the energy locked in a few of its atoms—was detonated at a height of 1,890 feet above the city. That bomb produced a temperature of 50 million degrees centigrade. Eighty thousand people were killed instantly or mortally wounded; 62,000 of the 90,000 buildings in Hiroshima were destroyed. Just three of the city's 55 hospitals and first-aid centers remained operable after the blast. 180 of the city's 200 doctors and 1,654 of its 1,780 nurses were dead or injured.

And all this came from releasing the energy locked in a few atoms. The energy in the atoms that make up our universe and body is incredibly powerful. It should never be underestimated.

Atoms Are the Elements
of Which Our World Is Made

Before universal intelligence could create life and human beings, it had to create the material world from which we would all be made. How did this happen?

Our earth is made up of 92 chemical elements. These are categorized in chemistry's Periodic Table, which tells us the composition of every one of these 92 elements. Each element is unique from the 91 others.

Incredibly, each of these atoms is made up of exactly the same three components. The first is called the *proton*. Protons carry a positive electrical charge. The second is the *neutron*, which

49

carries no charge at all. The third part of the atom is the *electron*, which carries a negative charge. The only difference between each of the 92 elements is the number of protons, neutrons and electrons in each.

By having different numbers of protons and electrons, each atom or element produces a different electromagnetic field. The information carried in its electromagnetic field determines what each atom will become. For instance, if an atom has 26 protons and electrons, it has the electromagnetic field that has the information to produce iron. If it has 79 protons and electrons, it has the electromagnetic field that forms gold.

Thus, every element or atom in our material world has been created and brought into existence by a specific electromagnetic field. Likewise, each human being is made up of the bioelectromagnetic information that created him or her. That information is our essence.

What Carries the Information of Life?

Since the information in our universe is carried by its electromagnetic waves, which waves carry the information that creates life?

The answer comes from Dr. Fritz-Albert Popp, a physicist from Munich, Germany. Dr. Popp's specialty is the study of biophotons. Photons are packages of energy, and bio means life. So biophotons are packages of the energy that carry the information of life.

Biophotons are made up of electromagnetic waves with a frequency range of 10^{14} to 10^{16} Hz (Hz = cycles per second) and they carry the information of life. All living things absorb photons of these frequencies. All living things also produce photons of this frequency. And when one cell of a living organism communicates with other cells, it does so by sending photons of this bioelectromagnetic frequency.

Popp further found that when any living organism died, the biophotons carrying bioelectromagnetic energy of 10^{14} to 10^{16}

Hz immediately and completely left the body. When that energy was gone, life ceased.

Obviously, these bioelectromagnetic frequencies are ubiquitous and essential to life. All of us are made up of the same 92 dead atoms or elements we've discussed above. They come alive when they are in the fields of bioelectromagnetic frequencies of 10^{14} to 10^{16} Hz. It is the information in these bioelectromagnetic waves that turns the "dead" elements into living elements.

Everything living is made up of cells that are composed of the life intelligence carried by these frequencies. They are the electromagnetic frequencies responsible for transporting the power, information and intelligence needed to create and maintain life! This is the energy we have to keep balanced for our bodies to be healthy.

How Do We Know Our Universe Was Created By and Consists of Universal Intelligence?

Dr. Popp's laboratory is the largest biophoton lab in the world. He proved the existence of bioelectromagnetic energy, and he determined which electromagnetic waves carry this information. He has instrumentation that will follow the path of a single biophoton in a living organism. From his extensive research, there can be no doubt which electromagnetic frequencies are the frequencies that create life.

But what about universal intelligence? It is not a measurable quantity. How do we know it exists and serves as the basis for life and growth?

To prove that an incredibly powerful intelligence fills our universe, you need only look at an acorn. Is there any chance it could have developed the intelligence and power and ability to become an oak tree by chance?

Impossible.

The intelligence of the energy that created and flows through an oak tree has to be available to it at all times. It has to be there

51

not only to create and design it, but to keep it alive. Just as each human being is unique, each oak tree is unique. To create and maintain such a complex, powerful thing without universal intelligence is illogical.

Universal intelligence works similarly to human intelligence. Think of one of those new cameras that self-focuses and exposes. If you point and shoot that camera you'll get a picture that is in focus and properly exposed. Does the camera have the knowledge to do this? Could the camera come into being by chance?

Impossible.

To test this, take all the materials out of which the camera is made—metal, glass, plastic, and so forth—in the exact amounts used to make the camera and put them in a blender. Then run the blender for one hour. Or one day. Or one week. Or one month. Even though all the parts of the camera are in the blender in the exact amounts and proportions, there is no possibility that the blender will produce a camera.

The point here is that the camera *required* human intelligence to first design it and manufacture it and finally use it to take a picture. In exactly the same way, your human body required an intelligence to design it, put it together and keep it living and functioning.

Compare the camera to the human eye. Each eye contains more than *1 billion working parts*. Light waves reflected from objects enter the eye. The lens of the eye automatically focuses that light on the retina of the eye, without any thinking or awareness on our part.

Likewise, the iris regulates the amount of light coming into the eye in much the same way as the camera does. *And it is automatic*. So is the retina, which is made up of photoreceptors. These photoreceptors consist of rods and cones that convert the mechanical light waves into a series of electrochemical codes that carry information to the brain. This means that each light wave carries not only color and brightness but also information.

52

Just like the biophotons Popp studied. The eye is an incredible, self-regulating mechanism. Nothing human intelligence has produced so far comes even close to the miracle of the eye. And the eye is only one part of the body.

You are made up of more than 100 trillion cells, each one a complete factory performing more than a million chemical reactions every second, day and night. Could these 100 trillion cells have come together by chance to form you? Could these 100 trillion cells perform 1 million chemical reactions a second perfectly, and perfectly interact with 100 trillion other cells by chance?

Not a chance.

When we interact with the universal creative energy inside our body—which is our essence—we bring the universal intelligence that created us into our lives. We become the envoy of our creator. This happens when we utilize the Biohealth System to interact with our essence

Biohealth Expands Your Life Into the Total World

It's important to point out again that Biohealth should not be seen as an alternative to medicine. It is more an *expansion* into the total world of the total body. Certainly, the material body that medicine ties itself to is of importance. But even more important is the world of energy and universal information and intelligence we've discussed in this chapter.

Much as the purpose of the universe is to evolve to higher states of intelligence, as is the purpose of humankind. Biohealth reminds us we live in a world in which we were designed to evolve to higher and higher levels of an ever increasing consciousness and awareness of both the material and nonmaterial aspects of our total world and total body.

The Biohealth student comes to realize that energy, or nonmaterial knowledge, is a matter of revelation. And our part, our purpose in life, is to be intellectually open to apprehend and comprehend that information as it is revealed to us. In this way, we are continually ready for new discoveries when they come. And come they will!

Still, there is one respect where humans don't operate like the universe. As far as we can tell, the universe continues to create and grow and evolve to higher states of intelligence with no real choice in the matter. Humans have a choice. The only way to maximize human evolution is by accessing universal information and intelligence you wouldn't be privy to without actively seeking it. You must choose to seek it!

The Biohealth System is a way to seek this kind of information and intelligence. It is a way to venture beyond the artificial barriers that traditional medicine and our own prejudices and preconceptions have constructed, and come to know the realities that exist beyond the material world of nature. The Biohealth System is a way to add universal knowledge to our lives, and by so doing evolve to higher levels of both consciousness and total health.

Beyond Your Limitations: Developing Your Personal Powers and Abilities

The view most people have of themselves and the reality they live in is both narrow and suffocating. They have a very limited perception of who they are and what they can become. They end up feeling inadequate and helpless. As a result, most people do not attain a healthy life.

Seeing themselves as powerless, they come to depend on others to solve their problems. They develop little personal power. They reduce themselves to lumps of matter and dismiss any notion they are composed of an incredible life energy of almost unlimited power.

Biohealth challenges this unreasonably low opinion of human potential. It refuses to surrender to the temptation to rely on experts with approved credentials to solve most of our prob-
54

lems for us. It takes serious issue with the belief that when any part of us ceases to function correctly, we are not an important part of restoring correct function.

Biohealth views each of us as having great personal power and inner resources. A major purpose of Biohealth is to rid ourselves of the belief that we are victims and empower us to see ourselves as a manifestation of an enormously powerful bioenergy, an energy that both created and maintains us.

We all have this incredibly powerful energy within us. We would not be alive if we didn't. The Biohealth System trains you to tune in to and use this energy in your daily life, and to reach your potential by accessing the universal information and intelligence that will help you evolve to your highest level of both consciousness and health.

When we rely entirely on others to solve our problems, even when they do solve them, we remain the same person who originally produced the problems. We have not become more than we were. We have not benefitted from the experience. Problems are opportunities for growth. They are chances to become more than we were before we had the problem. They are opportunities to incorporate more universal intelligence within ourselves.

In the Biohealth System you not only solve your problems, you transcend them. You use the problems of your own life to create a more powerful and wonderful you. Like the butterfly we discussed earlier, you develop your wings and become what you were created for and intended to be.

Much as the material and nonmaterial aspects of your body form one single organism, so the benefits of the Biohealth System simultaneously affect body, mind and spirit as the single unit they are. As such, the influence of the Biohealth System extends well beyond the confines of traditional medicine, our "material" body and our society's preference for "experts" and "credentials."

CHAPTER 4

Growing Younger as You Become Older– How Your Body Functions

There are no miracles because
ALL IS MIRACLE.
There is no magic because
ALL IS MAGIC.

—Llewelyn Powys, *A Pagan's Pilgrimage*

If you were to ask most people who or what they were, they'd probably point to their body and say, "This is me."

But is that really a good answer?

Modern research with "tagged" elements of the human body has shown that 98 percent of the atoms in your body are replaced by the body in less than a year. Like the universe, our bodies aren't static in nature. They are constantly changing.

The protein in your body is turned over every six months. You make an entirely new covering of skin every five weeks. You produce a new stomach lining *every five days!* Most of the functioning parts of your liver are replaced every six months.

Your skeleton every three months. The hydrogen, carbon, nitrogen and oxygen of your brain cells are replaced every year. The raw material of your DNA (the primary material in chromosomes and key to heredity and cell duplication) every six weeks.

It's incredible to think that when you meet a friend you haven't seen in six months, there is not one molecule in his or her face that was there the last time you saw him or her. Yet, some force has arranged all the new molecules in the same way as before. Although you're seeing an entirely new friend, at least physically, they can be recognized easily.

Look at a photograph of you at a year old. Then at five. Then 15. Then 25. Then 35. Then 45. Then 55. Then 65. Obviously, the person you see in each photo is very different, but they are all you. None of the photos you look at will be of the same human body, yet they are all photographs of you.

Every seven years, every cell of every part of your body dies and is replaced. Think of it! Over every seven-year period your physical body completely dies! Yet you live on! Every seven years you receive a completely new and older physical body.

What greater proof is there that you are more than your physical body? As each cell and every part of you dies, it is replaced by new cells and new parts that immediately become you and you alone. Therefore, you are not only created on the day you were conceived—you are being created and recreated every day of your life.

Biological health is based on the fact that you were not created at birth. All evidence indicates that you are continually being created. Birth is merely the initial step in the continuing process of being created. You are continually becoming more.

The physical "me" you point at today won't be the same "me" a few days from now. Yet, despite the constant changes, "you" remain "you." Clearly, to keep creating you and recreating you there must be something beyond the physical body at work. There must be an essence, an energy source, that is you and you alone.

58

How is this possible? The two laws of thermodynamics explain why this is not only possible but inevitable.

The Two Laws of Thermodynamics

As Albert Einstein once said, "The most incomprehensible thing about the universe is its comprehensibility." Contrary to what you may think when you're in a funk, the world out there is not all chaos. On the contrary. The universe and our lives operate under the rules of a very understandable set of laws.

Thermodynamics is the study of forms of energy and the conversion of these forms of energy into other forms. Its two laws go a long way toward showing us what we are, how we got here and where we are going. The Second Law of Thermodynamics says that every material entity in the universe that is a closed system (like a human body) and does work goes from an initial, highly organized state into a continually more disorganized state. The process of going from an organized to a disorganized state is called *entropy*. For anything living, it is called *aging*.

This law has a direct application to your body. After the age of 30, each year your physical body becomes more "disorganized." It loses strength and fitness. Its metabolism slows down. Ultimately the disorder of our body system becomes so great that it can no longer function. This is death, which is simply our body obeying the Second Law.

But what of that unique bioenergy called our "essence"? The energy that created and defines us. Does it die, too? This is where the First Law of Thermodynamics comes in. Our essence is bioenergy. The First Law states that energy can neither be created nor destroyed. It can only be transformed. Therefore, our essence, which is energy, cannot be destroyed. What then happens to our bioenergy self, our essence? The first law tells us—it is transformed.

How is our bioenergy transformed? Our mind is a function of our essence. Our essence and mind function as one unit, a mind-essence.

How We Grow Younger as We Grow Older

The mind function of our essence is continually adding information. Therefore our mind-essence is continually becoming more complicated, which by the laws of thermodynamics means it is getting younger. By these laws, the more disorganized anything has become, the older it is. The more organized it is, the more complicated and younger it is. Whatever is becoming more disorganized is becoming older, Whatever is becoming more organized, more complicated, is becoming younger.

By these two laws our human body reaches its youngest at about the ages of 25 and 30, and then gets older until it can no longer function. Although our physical body gets more disorganized, our energy body—our essence-mind—takes in more information and becomes more organized and more complex, which means it becomes younger. By using our mind to bring in more and more information, as our material body becomes disorganized and eventually is dead, our essence becomes transformed to a more complicated form and becomes younger.

The objective of life on earth is that when our physical body has died, our youngest possible essence passes on. The Biohealth System, by keeping your physical body at its youngest for the longest possible time and by adding information to your essence, helps you to achieve this objective.

Some Thoughts on Death

I don't really like the term "death." When somebody I know "dies" I simply say he or she has "passed on." The First Law dictates that energy, which our essence is, cannot be destroyed. What waits for our essence next, I can't tell you. Nobody knows.

What then is "death"? I know what death is for me. For me death is a command to live every day to its fullest. Period.

Energy Research

I hope the previous explanation will help you understand and realize that equating existence with your temporary body is a mistake. When you create a conceptual idea that you are your physical body it ultimately becomes reality for you. Then, when your body functions incorrectly, you try to correct the body instead of the energy source responsible for creating the malfunction. You end up treating a separate body part or symptom instead of the root cause of the problem.

With the Biohealth System, you communicate not only with the chemicals of your physical body but directly with the life energy that created you and controls body function. Skeptics will claim this energy doesn't exist. They will say it's a product of my own imagination or entirely hypothetical and unsupported by research.

They're wrong. What follows is an overview of research on bioenergy done by two highly respected scientists, an anatomist and physicist, Harold Saxton Burr and Fritz-Albert Popp. Both work within the rigid prove-it mentality of the scientific method and both have found, through their research, that bioenergy is the source of life and health.

Dr. Harold Saxton Burr

Harold Saxton Burr, PhD, was a member of the Yale University School of Medicine for 43 years teaching gross anatomy and neuroanatomy to his students. During that time, he published more than 93 scientific papers. Along with teaching, Burr researched extensively on what he called the "electric patterns" of life.

After his retirement—as E. K. Hunt, professor of anatomy emeritus at Yale—in order to prove that man is a bioelectromagnetic field he wrote his classic, breakthrough book

61

Blueprint for Immortality. This book is required reading for anyone wishing to understand the meaning of life. The following quotes are from this book.

At the top of Burr's achievements was the discovery that bioenergy—or electrodynamic fields, as he called them—maintained and controlled all life. He was one of the first people to both prove and quantify the existence of bioenergy with his own instrumentation. In *Immortality* he concludes that, "Man—and, in fact, *all* forms (of life)—are ordered and controlled by electro-dynamic fields which can be measured and mapped with precision." Wow.

These electrodynamic fields are "basic with the necessary power and directional properties to determine the processes inherent in the growth and development of any living system." Since the "electrodynamic" fields Burr measured were clearly the fields on which life depended, he ended up naming them *L-fields*, short for "life fields." The "organizing and directing" qualities of these L-Fields" were confirmed by Burr in thousands of experiments.

Until Burr came along, biologists had no explanation for the ability of the body to maintain itself through ceaseless metabolic and material changes. It was a mystery to them. But Burr found that electrodynamic fields in the body served as a "matrix or mould" that preserved it. Burr was the first to show scientifically why you are the same you at age one and age 70—you don't have the same body, but you both have the same L-field.

For instance, Burr found that by examining the L-field in a frog's egg electrically, he could show the future location of the frog's nervous system. "This is because the frog's L-field is the matrix which will determine the form which will develop from the egg," he explained. As such, Burr determined that his L-fields were not only necessary to maintenance and the constant re-creation of the body but the actual, original form of the being as well.

Dr. Burr was also able to diagnose disease by changes in L-fields in much the same way we do in the Biohealth System. There were even applications to psychiatry. Dr. Leonard J. Ravitz, a psychiatrist who worked with Dr. Burr, discovered that changes in L-fields could indicate a subject's psychological condition. When a person was excited and felt "on top of the world," his or her L-field voltages measured high. When people felt confused, puzzled or "below par," their voltages measured correspondingly low. By reading L-fields, Dr. Ravitz claimed he could determine which psychiatric hospital patients should be released and which required continued treatment.

Another finding of Burr—and one very important to Biohealth—was that while each part (entity) of the body was important, "the relationship of the entities were quite as important as the entities themselves." This emphasis on the whole body and the relationship between its parts both material and non-material is at the core of Biohealth today.

Burr also questioned the reliance on biochemistry embraced by modern medicine. "To be sure the chemistry is of great importance because this is the gasoline that makes the buggy go," he wrote. "But the chemistry of a living system does not determine the functional properties of a living system any more than changing the gas makes a Rolls-Royce out of a Ford."

It was important to Burr that his research not be seen as merely theoretical. He knew how resistant people could be to new and original thought and how important "hard" science was to proving his case. That's why all his findings were based on exhaustive measurement and research. Every statement in Burr's *Immortality* book, for instance, is substantiated by research findings. This was a man who did his homework.

But perhaps the most important legacy of Burr's work comes in its application to our principle of "essence." By proving the existence of individual bioelectromagnetic fields or bioenergy, he also opened the door to the revelation that, as the First Law of Thermodynamics would predict, we don't "die." He felt strongly enough about this to title his major work, *Blueprint for Immortality*. Pure energy, like our essence, does not age, nor is it destroyed. It is transformed and passes on.

Again, this fits very well into the Biohealth System philosophy.

More on Dr. Popp

In the last chapter we briefly discussed Dr. Fritz-Albert Popp's work with biophotons, or packages of life energy. Dr. Popp found that all living organisms absorb and emit biophotons and that these biophotons disappear upon death of the body.

Popp also found that in the human body DNA takes up biophotons, stores them and serves as the source for biophoton emission. In this way, as has now been confirmed by genetic research, DNA controls the biochemical and physiological reactions of every cell.

DNA does this by sending out instructions to the cell through RNA. How does it do this? Popp's studies show that the RNA produced by DNA is the direct result of photons, or the bioenergy, it has absorbed.

This, in turn, has a great effect on biochemistry and physiology. If the biophotons (or bioelectromagnetic fields) are correct, the DNA will keep the body functioning correctly. If they're not, the DNA will send out faulty messages and the body will function incorrectly. Thus, it's not the biochemicals produced that are the basic cause of illness but the incorrect information sent to cells resulting from an imbalanced, deficient bioelectromagnetic field pattern.

Whereas Dr. Burr's research was done mostly in the 1930s and 1950s, Dr. Popp's research is state of the art. I took a workshop with him in Munich in 1985 and his lectures and demonstrations changed my life.

Popp's aim during our time together was to demonstrate how communication occurs between organisms by means of electromagnetic fields. Using a photon multiplier as a chief measuring instrument, he convincingly showed us time and time again that every cell in your body communicates with every other cell by means of electromagnetic radiation.

The title of Dr. Popp's 1979 book, *Electromagnetic Bio-Information*, is very instructive. It describes the focus of Popp's work—that biological and physiological information is communicated by the cells of living organisms through electromagnetic radiation, or bioelectromagnetic field patterns. These field patterns, by the way, are the same field patterns we tune in to in the Biohealth System.

To study this phenomenon, Dr. Popp analyzed signals coming from living systems to look for correlations between these signals and biological and physiological functions. All of the following quotations are from the Popp lecture of April 22, 1985. He found that "photon emission is correlated to all biological functions within the organisms, and to all biochemical reactions." In other words, bioelectromagnetic radiation controls our physiological and biological functions. He also found that photons were capable of, and were the only force available for, regulating the millions of reactions that take place in a cell during a mere second's time.

Popp's continuing research keyed on the cellular communication provided by photons. He called them the "base for communication of the cells between each other." This communication system comprised the "most fundamental base of communication" in the body because it worked "between cells, between all the single systems of cells."

He also found that photons were "coherent radiation." This means they radiated laser beams. They could thus work between all single systems of cells at the highest speed possible—the speed of light. What's more, they had a higher "coherence," or constituted a much more "refined technical system" than the lasers we can produce with our advanced technology. While industrial lasers emit only limited wavelengths, the biological system emits an infinite number of wavelengths!

Dr. Popp further discovered that this advanced bioenergy communication system was at fault during disease. Cancer cells, which grow wild and destroy cells rather than cooperate, "lost the possibility of taking up mutual photons from each other." When cells failed to communicate, disease resulted. When cell cooperation is restored, so is health.

Popp's research adds strong, scientific support to Biohealth's focus on bioelectromagnetic fields. Popp proved that bioelectromagnetic radiation controlled biological function, communicated biologic and physiologic information and that the root cause of disease and incorrect function was not biochemistry but the bioenergy that created it.

He also took his work with the body on to universal applications, much as Biohealth does. "We are pictures of our external world," he said. "Our external world is an electromagnetic field pattern. Look at the sunlight. Look at the optical signals we receive. You can make what you like of it, but always you will find an electromagnetic interaction. So we are in a sea of electromagnetic influences. And these influences can be stored in some substances. And fortunately the substances with the highest storage capacity for these signals are biological materials!"

We are, thus, as our universe is, primarily electromagnetic. And as Dr. Popp, Dr. Burr and many others have shown, we are much more than our physical bodies. Each of us possesses a unique, individualized electromagnetic field pattern. When our electromagnetic energies are at proper strength and balance, our bodies function perfectly. When our electromagnetic fields are distorted, our bodies produce the wrong chemicals and function incorrectly, leading to numerous health problems.

The Biohealth System strives to make you the master of these electromagnetic field patterns and, by so doing, live your life at its highest, most successful, most productive level. When your physical body is no more, we want your youngest possible essence to pass on. With our initial questions about the nature, source and purpose of life now answered, we'll examine the blueprint for the Biohealth System itself in the next chapter.

CHAPTER 5

The Biohealth System— Test and Grow Healthy!

*Nothing in the world is so difficult as to free
the mind of prejudice and preconception.*

—Llewelyn Powys, *The Pathetic Fallacy*

How important is your health to you?

How important is it to wake up in the morning feeling fit, confident and capable of being your best for the day to come?

How important is it to be free of the worry and loss of energy, productivity and confidence that come with ill health?

How important would it be if I told you that there is a way to know how healthy you are without doubt, doctors or intrusive medical testing?

Or that there was a way to return many weak or diseased parts of your body to healthy function without drugs or surgery?

Or that you could experience total wellness?

The Biohealth System shows you how to achieve this and, without any fanfare or office visits, gets you started achieving it right now.

You don't need a degree or credentials to use the Biohealth System. Or any vague, technical, medical language or explanations. The principle behind Biohealth is really quite simple: *Health and disease in your body are determined by your biomagnetic fields.* When the biomagnetic field of any part of your body is properly balanced it functions correctly and produces health. When the biomagnetic field of any part of you is not balanced, it cannot function correctly and illness results.

It's that simple.

The Biohealth Window

The Biohealth System is built on giving you a window through which you can look into your body, see each organ and its biomagnetic field and determine if it's balanced. Even more exciting, when you look through that window and identify an imbalanced biomagnetic field, the Biohealth instruction book you're now reading (and your own body) will tell you what you need to do to restore it to the balanced, correct state that produces health.

Then, when you've restored balance to that biomagnetic field, you use the Biohealth window to show you what you need to do to keep it balanced and your body functioning at its best.

Finally, you use that window to prove that what you have done has restored biological health. When your body itself, without outside help, is achieving and maintaining balanced biomagnetic fields, you have biological health. Biological health is the goal of the Biohealth System. By using your Biohealth window, you will know when you've achieved it.

And that's another big part of the Biohealth System: proof.

It is a law in the Biohealth System that you believe nothing until you prove it. You prove that your body has health only when you determine that your body itself, with only your own lifestyle and diet as support, is producing balanced biomagnetic fields.

Biohealth is noninvasive. It can do no harm. Where X-rays provide, at best, a two-dimensional shadow of a three-dimensional object, the Biohealth window actually allows you to "see" how each part of your body is working.

Perhaps best of all, the Biohealth System doesn't require that you put your precious health in another person's hands. You do it yourself. You take charge. Where the doctor is involved, it puts you in the driver's seat by giving you a way to monitor what he's doing and make sure you're getting the results *you* want.

The Seven-Step Biohealth System Program

The Biohealth System is basically about electricity. Moving magnetic fields produce electric currents to run the machines at a factory or boot your computer at work or light the lights in your home. They do the same kind of work inside your body.

Every magnetic field in your body produces an electric current. Because we are dealing with a living being (you) we call the fields, which produce the current *bio*electromagnetic. For the sake of brevity, we refer to them also as "biomagnetic" or "bioenergy" fields.

The entire Biohealth System is based on the fact that when you have balanced biomagnetic fields your body produces the correct chemistry and correct electricity for healthy function. With bioenergy balance the body's muscles (machines), computer (brain), lights (senses) and all its other parts work perfectly and do the job they're supposed to do. The goal of the Biohealth System is to keep those biomagnetic (bioenergy) fields balanced and your body working at peak performance levels.

The following seven-step guide to the Biohealth System will give you a preview of what you will be doing when you begin the program itself in Chapter 10. As you work through chapters 10 through 13, you will perform each of these steps in pursuit of Biohealth's goal: your biological health.

Step 1–Testing

This involves the specially designed Biohealth testing magnet. The testing magnet allows you to test and "see" each biomagnetic field in your body. The test magnet is, basically, a "window" into yourself. If each organ of your body has balanced bioenergy, correct function will be produced in the organ and this, in turn, will produce health. If an organ is found to be imbalanced, that means it cannot function correctly and it is open to disease. In this case, the testing magnet takes on a whole new job, which we'll describe in step 4.

Step 2–Restoring Bioenergy Balance

There is another kind of magnet you use in the Biohealth System called an "energy balancing magnet" or "correcting magnet." It is used to balance an imbalanced magnetic field and provide an environment where organs can heal and return to proper function.

The correcting magnet works because all of your body organs are *paramagnetic*, which means that when you put the organ in the field of a magnet, the organ assumes the strength and polarity of that magnet. The correcting magnets you will use are of the proper strength so that, when placed over an organ where a magnetic field is out of balance, the magnetic energy in short supply (north or south) will be increased to the point that it is in balance. Through the paramagnetic properties of the body's organs, the correcting magnet is able to balance the organ's biomagnetic field to proper proportions.

It's important to say here that the balancing magnet doesn't do it all. In fact, it's not really responsible for getting you healthier. It simply creates an environment in which healing and health can occur. The reason you balance the bioenergy field of an organ is because the organ functions better when the bioenergy fields are balanced. You balance the biomagnetic field with the correcting magnet so the organ will have the strength to restore its health.

As long as the field is in an imbalanced state, the organ cannot function correctly. It can't produce enough energy to do its job. It can't take in nutrition either. You can eat the best foods but you won't properly assimilate and metabolize them without bioenergy balance. Indeed, nutrition is meaningless without energy balance. This energy balance is the gift the balancing magnet gives to the organ.

Without the magnet, the organ doesn't metabolize food properly and doesn't produce enough energy for healing. It is under oxidative stress, which means the organ will never have enough electrons to do its job or, more precisely, produce the correct electric current to do the job it's supposed to do.

As soon as you put the correcting magnet over an unbalanced organ, the organ begins to assimilate food and produce the right electric current and energy. Healing begins immediately and continues through what is usually a three- to four-month period before the organ can maintain correct function by itself (see step 7).

Technically, when your body produces a balanced state itself without outside help it has achieved biological health. When the balancing magnet is used, we call the energy produced *magnetic bioenergy*, since an outside agent (the magnet) is responsible for the energy balance. Our goal in the Biohealth System is to get your own body balancing your bioenergy. When your body does this, you have biological health. Only at this point do you have true Biohealth.

Step 3—Stopping the Autoimmune Attack

When an organ has an unbalanced bioenergy field and is not functioning correctly, the body begins to see the organ as a foreign substance and produces antibodies to attack it. In this situation the body, basically, is attacking itself. This is called an "autoimmune" attack.

For healing to take place, we must stop the autoimmune attack of the body on its own organs by diverting the antibodies.

We do this by taking a substance called a protomorphogen (PMG). A PMG is a small piece of the same organ under attack in your body taken from an animal.

For example, if you had a diseased prostate you would ingest a piece of animal prostate in tablet form. The antibodies that were attacking your prostate would then begin to attack the animal prostate in the tablet you've taken. Antibodies are tissue specific but not species specific, so they don't care what kind of prostate they attack as long as it's a prostate. They are thus diverted to the PMG. The autoimmune attack on your prostate ends and the prostate is given time to heal.

In the Biohealth System, when you place a correcting magnet over a malfunctioning organ you also use the PMG of that organ. As long as the correcting magnet is indicated, you need the PMG to defend yourself against autoimmune attacks. When biological health is achieved in step 7 you will no longer need the magnet or the PMG.

Step 4—Determining the Correct Nutrition for You

The testing magnet you used in step 1 is used for another purpose here. In order for healing to occur and health to be maintained, you must give your body the food—and sometimes supplements—it needs. Since every person has unique needs, this can involve some serious guesswork.

Unless you're using the Biohealth System.

By using the test magnet, there is no guessing. The test magnet determines what foods and supplements your body needs. With the test magnet, before you put anything in your body, you determine if it is right for it. *The test magnet allows you to test how well anything will work before you take or use it!*

With your Biohealth window—the test magnet—you will see what effect anything will have on your biomagnetic energy *before* you take it. With the test magnet there's no need to worry about doing harm to your body by taking or doing the wrong thing. It replaces guessing with fact. *You* have control where none existed before. You have the knowledge, information and power to give your body what it needs for healthy functioning. This is a very important tool in achieving health.

But the substance testing program doesn't work alone. While taking the correct supplements and food are critical to your success, it is equally important that they be digested and assimilated. Remember what we said earlier. No matter how good your foods, if you have unbalanced energy and an organ undergoing an autoimmune attack, your body won't be able to fully digest and assimilate the food you take regardless of its quality.

Balancing bioenergy by itself is not enough. Stopping the autoimmune attack by itself is not enough. Eating the right foods by itself is not enough. All three are required!

Steps 2 through 4 work together in the Biohealth System. To digest and metabolize the foods you eat, you must have bioenergy balance and you must stop any autoimmune attack. Only when this is done are you able to fully metabolize the foods and supplements you take and become and remain healthy.

Step 5—Applying and Monitoring the Biohealth Program

In step 5 your test magnet becomes a monitoring magnet. By monitoring we mean you test each area of biomagnetic imbalance until your test magnet shows you that it is now balanced. You continue to monitor the health of your body as you apply the program and you keep monitoring it until the bioenergy fields are balanced and symptoms have been removed.

At this point you have achieved balance and health but it might not be enough. If your health continues to depend on wearing magnets or taking PMGs, you do not have biological health. You have synthetic health. To ensure that you have biological health, that you are producing biomagnetic energy, you must prove it.

Step 6—Proving the Program

How do you prove biological health? The only way to prove it is to move your body deliberately into a state of imbalanced bioenergy and see if your body itself can return the imbalance to proper balance and function.

We'll tell you more about how this is done later in the book but, at its simplest, what we do is use our correcting magnet to create an imbalanced state in the organ in question. As soon as you've created an imbalance you take the magnet and the PMG away. If you have biological health your body will return the organ to balanced bioenergy without the use of a correcting magnet or a PMG, usually within two to four weeks.

At that point, you've proven that your body can achieve and maintain balanced bioenergy fields. You have also proven that you have biological health.

If the organ remains imbalanced, you know you have more work to do.

Step 7—Maintaining Correct Function

The purpose of the Biohealth System is not only to restore correct function and health, but to keep it that way. You do that by using your test magnet to continually monitor your bioenergy fields, the foods you eat, supplements you take and indeed, your entire lifestyle. In the Biohealth System, your goal is not only to test and grow healthy! It's to test and stay healthy!

This is a very important point. As your life situation changes, so do your needs. By monitoring the changes going on in your body you can determine what is needed to keep your bioenergy fields in balance and your body functioning correctly. Biohealth is much more than getting you healthy. It is about keeping you healthy.

Life is a dynamic process. Therefore, you need a dynamic program to maintain health. The perfect program is one that allows you to continue monitoring your health while continuing to monitor what your body needs.

This is precisely what the Biohealth System does.

In a time of drastic change it is the learners who inherit the future. The learned usually find themselves equipped to live in a world that no longer exists.

—Eric Hoffer

What you honor is what you will cultivate.

—Sanford C. Frumker

CHAPTER 6

What Is Magnetism?

We are licensed to spend our days as we desire,
gathering our experiences as a stranger gathers
shells at the margin of the sea.

—Llewelyn Powys, *Now That the Gods Are Dead*

Magnetism is an unseen, untouchable energy that comes from magnets. Energy, by definition, is the capacity to do work. Therefore, magnetic energy is the ability of magnets to do work. We will talk about the work magnets do in this chapter. Through this discussion you'll get an introduction to the potential of magnets, their effect on living tissue and a background on how the testing and correcting magnets used in the Biohealth System do the things they do.

The Basics

Every magnet has two poles: a north pole at one end or side and a south pole at the other end or side. Opposite magnetic poles attract each other. Like magnetic poles repel each other. If you put the south pole of one magnet near the north pole of another magnet, the two will attract each other and join together. If you place the south poles of two magnets or the north poles of two magnets near each other, they will repel each other and move apart.

The magnetic field of a magnet is the area around the north or south pole that is affected by the magnetism. It is the area in which the force of the magnetic energy is exerted, the area in which it does its work. In the Biohealth System, the organ being tested or balanced is in the magnetic field of the testing or correcting magnet.

One of the great things about magnetic energy is that it will go through almost any substance without being weakened. This insures the success of our testing and correcting magnets in the Biohealth System. Skin and body tissue offer no resistance to magnetic energy. Magnetic energy does its job without body barriers.

Magnetic energy is, however, rapidly weakened by distance. As you move away from a magnet the strength of its magnetic field rapidly decreases. The effect of a magnet close to a substance may be substantial but, at a distance, the same magnet may have no effect at all.

The strength of a magnet is measured in *gauss*. This term was coined in honor of nineteenth-century German mathematician Karl Friedrich Gauss who performed early experiments with electromagnetism. Gauss measures magnetic energy. The greater the gauss, the stronger the magnet and the stronger the magnetic field it produces. The lower the gauss, the weaker the magnet and the weaker its magnetic field.

The strength of magnetic fields varies widely. The earth's magnetic field measures only about 0.5 gauss. A cyclotron, a device used to accelerate electric particles to very high energy, may have a strength of 20,000 gauss. The test magnet we use in the Biohealth System is 1,000 gauss. The correcting magnet around 3,700 gauss.

It is important to understand the relation of electricity to magnetism. As discussed earlier, every electric current produces a magnetic field perpendicular to it. Every time a magnetic field varies, it produces an electric field. Electricity and magnetism are thus two aspects of the same force. We do not deal with an electric force or a magnetic force when using magnets. We deal with an electromagnetic force.

The Flow of Magnetic Energy

We all live on a magnet called Earth. As all magnets it has a north and south pole. In using the Biohealth System, it is important to understand that philosophically these two poles are completely different. They are, in every sense, the opposite of each other.

Take a look at the illustration below of a 6-inch magnetic bar. It has a north pole at one end and a south pole at the other. Magnetic energy between the poles travels from south to north and back again but it does not travel directly. Nor does it flow in the same direction from each pole.

How Magnetic Energy Flows

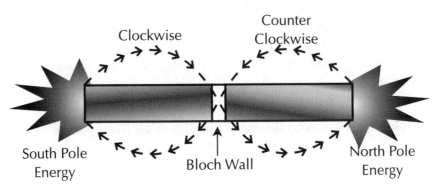

Energy from the south pole moves in a clockwise direction (see illustration) to the middle of the bar where it passes through the magnet and emerges on the opposite side of the bar. When it emerges from the opposite side it now travels toward the north pole in a counterclockwise direction.

When the magnetic energy arrives at the north pole, it continues to move in a counterclockwise direction. But when it again reaches the middle of the bar, it again crosses over at the Bloch wall to the other side. When it emerges from the opposite side, it is traveling in a clockwise direction again and moving toward the south pole.

The direct center of the magnet through which the magnetic energy flows and changes its direction is a point of zero magnetism. This crossover area, this area of zero magnetism, is called the bloch wall.

How Magnetic Energy Flows

The magnetic energy of the south pole half of the magnet moves in a clockwise direction. The energy of the north pole half moves in a counterclockwise direction. The two magnetic energies are opposites. Most importantly to Biohealth, they also affect your body in opposite ways.

The Effects of the Two Magnetic Poles on Living Systems

Serendipity can play a big role in science and research. Indeed, the discovery by Dr. Albert Roy Davis that the two magnetic poles change and alter biological systems in opposite ways was made by total accident. Davis and Walter C. Rawls tell the story in their book *Magnetism and Its Effects on the Living System*.

Dr. Davis enjoyed fishing. One day in 1936 he placed three boxes of worms in cardboard containers on his workbench in preparation for an upcoming fishing expedition. Also on that workbench was a horseshoe magnet and Davis, without thinking about it, just happened to place one box on the north pole of the magnet, one box on the south pole and one box at a distance from the magnet.

The next morning, Davis arrived to make a stunning discovery. The worms on the south pole had eaten through the side of the container, a feat of no small strength and will. Dr. Davis wondered if the poles of the magnet might have had something to do with this so he decided to test this theory. He got heavier containers for the earthworms and this time quite deliberately placed one container on the south pole of a magnet, one on the north and one away from the magnets for a period of 12 days.

What he found was astonishing. The worms on the south pole grew to be one-third larger than the worms not on a magnet. They were longer in length and diameter and extremely active. A number of babies had also been born.

The north pole produced opposite results. Many of the earthworms had died and those still alive were thin and showed little activity. The third box, the control group of worms, showed no changes or differences either way.

Further tests confirmed the totally opposite results obtained by placing worms on different magnetic poles. South pole worms were found to experience a sharp rise in their protein amino acids which led to an increase in physical strength and development. Meanwhile, north pole worms experienced an actual loss of protein amino acids leading to lower physical strength and development.

The Magnetic Exposure of Seeds

Davis's original studies were followed up by hundreds of other experiments conducted to measure the effect of magnetic exposure on seeds.

It was found that seeds treated with the south pole of a magnet before planting produced larger plants. Those treated with the north pole produced smaller plants. The south pole plants also showed a rise in temperature and an increase in carbon dioxide intake. They also liberated more oxygen and the length and size of their roots were greater.

The north pole plants went in the opposite direction. Overall, the south pole plants increased life, growth and development. The north pole plants arrested life, growth and development.

How did magnetic energy achieve these effects? Another experiment done with tomato seeds gives us a big clue. Many people cannot eat tomatoes because of their acidity. It was thought that magnetic energy might affect acidity in the tomato and make it more palatable to a wider range of people.

This belief led to an exciting research project. South-pole–treated tomato seeds produced a more acid tomato. The north-pole–treated seeds did produce a less acid variety.

More importantly, it was found that there were no changes in the chemical content of the tomatoes as a result of the magnetic fields. There were changes in acidity but not in the biochemistry of the tomato or seed. With no biochemical changes found, the change in acidity had to come as a result of a change in genetic function. Thus, magnetic energy applied to seeds actually changed the function of their genes. The south pole stimulated genetic function to increase life, growth and development. The north pole weakened genetic function so that it arrested life, growth and development.

North and South Pole Effects on Small Animals

Even greater evidence of the differing effects of the two poles on life systems came in research on hens and roosters. South-pole–treated chicks grew faster and stronger than north pole chicks. They also ate more than north pole chicks.

But with these physical effects came some rather severe psychological and behavioral effects. The resulting intelligence of the physically stronger south pole chickens measured lower than their counterparts. Even more remarkable, the south pole roosters in the last stages of maturity became cannibalistic and ate the flesh of hens of their own kind. They would mount the backs of other birds and peck, scratch and dig until they killed them.

Along with the aggression and arrested intelligence, south pole animals also exhibited an indifference to their surroundings. Their cages were filthy. North pole chickens were, by comparison, neat and clean and sensitive to their surroundings.

Thus, the effects of single pole energy on the chicks presented a truly mixed bag. Advantages were negated by disadvantages. Single pole energy provided one-dimensional animals and a lack of balance in physical and behavioral characteristics. Overall, south pole energy made the chicks stronger and more aggressive but also less intelligent and aware. North pole energy hindered physical development but created neater and smarter chicks.

Obviously, balance gave the ideal result.

Effects on Mice and Rats

Much the same effects were found with mice and rats when exposed to north and south pole magnetic energy. South pole mothers were stronger and delivered their babies with less effort. Newborn south pole babies developed faster and were stronger in every respect than control group rodents.

The opposite was true for north pole babies. They developed slower than controls and were weaker. North pole babies were also smaller than controls and north pole mothers weaker.

But, as with the chicks, south pole mice and rats performed little maintenance on their cages and seemed content to sleep in their own mire and filth. North pole rats and mice, on the other hand, took a great deal of time to wash themselves and keep their cages and nests clean.

It was also found that the life span of rodents and other animals could be extended up to 50 percent by applying the south pole intrauterine at the first stages of development. This again showed the ability of magnetic energy to alter gene function.

The north pole animals also showed an extended life span, but for a very different reason. Their increased life span was due to a change in genetic function that slowed down their metabolism. Basically, slowing the animals' growth to maturity led to a longer life span.

Interestingly, when the south pole was applied to mice and rats *after* birth it shortened their life span for much the same reason. An excessive increase in metabolism led to a much earlier death.

It should be noted that, like the hens and roosters above, the north pole mice and rats were more intelligent than their muscle-bound, slow-to-learn south pole counterparts.

Over 300 similar experiments were performed in an eight year period. Further information on findings can be located in the book *Magnetism and Its Effects on the Living System*. We also recommend Davis and Rawls' book, *The Magnetic Effect*. There is excellent material in these two books on the use of magnetic energy to control cancers and tumors, nerve pain and many other conditions.

These findings held great importance for the Biohealth System. Clearly, too much north pole or south pole energy had extreme effects on genetic function. A balance between the two would be necessary for optimal health and well-being. As such, balanced bioenergy produced physical and mental health.

The following is a review of the effects of north pole magnetic energy:

- The north pole magnetic energy vasoconstricts (closes down) blood vessels. The north pole thus controls bleeding and speeds up the coagulation of blood.

- The north pole provides a sedative reaction and helps control pain. It has proven especially helpful in controlling pain from burns.

- The north pole slows down organ activity. It also slows down overactive organs, inflammation and trauma. By producing a counterclockwise spin in the DNA and making the nucleus spin counterclockwise, activity and the effects of injury are slowed by north pole energy.

- The north pole thus brings oxygen into the tissue but it never produces the oxidized free radicals that contribute to cell malfunction.

- The north pole fights infection. Microorganisms are retarded by north pole energy. The oxygen north pole energy brings to the tissue is also destructive to microorganisms and parasites.

- The north pole attracts extracellular fluid. If a tissue is injured and edematous (filled with fluid) the north pole can be placed a small distance from the edematous tissue to pull the fluid out of the edematous tissue and limit swelling and pain. If the north pole is placed over edematous tissue, however, it will increase the fluid and pain.

- The north pole removes hydrogen ions and produces a less acidic and more alkaline tissue. To function correctly, any part of the body must have the correct number of hydrogen ions, which are electrically charged atoms. When hydrogen ions are in excess, the organ is too acidic and energy is drained away instead of produced. North pole energy can correct for this situation and bring hydrogen ions to the correct level. (See the next chapter.)

- The north pole increases potassium ions in the tissue. Potassium plays a role in changing food into energy and new tissue, and aids the flow of fluid to cells of the body.

- The north pole reduces the amount of inorganic calcium deposits in the body. It dissolves calcium deposits around arthritic joints.

- The north pole reduces fatty deposits. This is because fatty deposits are acidic and the north pole removes the hydrogen ions responsible for acidity. This is a slow process, however.

- The north pole can shrink tumors and arrest cancer (we'll discuss this further in Chapter 13).

- The north pole can increase mental alertness.

The following is a review of the effects of south pole magnetic energy:

- South pole magnetic energy causes vasodilation, which expands the size of blood vessels and blood flow.

- South pole magnetic energy increases the number of hydrogen ions, thus increasing acidity in the tissue. This can improve all forms of digestion.

- By expanding the size of blood vessels, the south pole produces a greater flow of fluids. When placed on an edematous area, it disperses excess fluid and can lessen pain and swelling.

- Placed over the thymus, an important gland in the upper chest/lower neck area, the south pole increases immune system action.

- The south pole increases protein activity.

- The south pole increases sodium. Sodium plays a role in tissue formation and the flow of fluid into body cells.

- South pole energy stimulates any tissue on which it is placed. This promotes growth and strength, though it's important to realize that growth and strength are not always a good thing for health. For instance, the south pole should never be placed on a tumor or cancer because it will energize them and make them more powerful. Likewise, the south pole should never be placed on an infection because it will strengthen the infecting bacteria.

As shown previously, south pole (also called *positive)* and north pole (also called *negative)* magnetic energies have opposite effects when applied to living systems. Of and by itself, each pole can produce conditions harmful to your health. Each can also produce beneficial effects.

The key here is balance. When north and south pole energies are in balance they produce a magnetic bioenergy balance that also produces correct function and health. When a tissue or organ is out of balance to the north pole we use the magnetic south pole of a correcting magnet to balance it. When it is out of balance to the south pole we use the magnetic north pole to balance it.

We'll see how this principle is properly used in the Biohealth training chapters to follow. It's important to understand the importance of the hydrogen ion and pH (acidity-alkalinity) in creating the balanced bioenergy we're in search of. This information lays the foundation for the whole Biohealth System.

CHAPTER 7

The Hydrogen Ion and pH

Let us use wisdom where wisdom may be used,
but ultimately let us be obedient to destiny, to
our own destiny, seeking it out as a young gull
seeks the sea.

—Llewelyn Powys, *Impassioned Clay*

As you may recall from our discussion in Chapter 3, every material thing is made of atoms. The chair you sit on, the food you eat, the air you breathe, your own body—they're all made up of atoms.

The atom consists of three types of particles—protons, electrons and neutrons. Protons carry a positive electric charge. Neutrons carry no charge. Electrons carry a negative charge.

At the center of every atom is a nucleus. The nucleus is made up of protons and neutrons. The hydrogen atom has a single proton in its nucleus. All others have multiple protons. These protons attract electrons which are in an orbit around the nucleus.

Neutrons in the nucleus provide a strong force for binding protons together. Remember that like charges repel each other.

Since protons all have positive charges, they should repel each other and the atom fly apart. Thanks to neutrons, they don't. There are an equal number of neutrons and protons in the nucleus and these neutrons bind protons together so they remain bunched in the nucleus.

Outside the nucleus in the body of the atom, is the same number of electrons as there are protons. Each proton has a positive charge and each electron a negative charge. Since the number of electrons equals the number of protons, the number of positive charges equals the number of negative charges and the atom itself has no charge.

What Is an Ion? What Is a Hydrogen Ion?

Remember, again from our discussion in Chapter 3, that the number of protons in an atom produces different magnetic fields. These different magnetic fields produce different atoms. If an atom has 20 protons the magnetic field it produces makes a calcium atom. The magnetic field produced by 79 protons makes a gold atom. The magnetic field of a single proton produces hydrogen.

An atom cannot gain or lose a proton. If it did, it would become a different atom. However, electrons are very light and move easily. Atoms can easily gain and lose electrons and still be the same atom.

When an atom gains an electron it has a negative charge. When it loses an electron it has a positive charge. When an atom gains or loses an electron and becomes positively or negatively charged it is called an *ion*. An ion is an atom with an electrical charge.

Since hydrogen has only one proton, it is the only atom without a neutron. Having only one proton, it has no need of neutrons to bind protons together. When it loses its electron, only the proton remains leaving the hydrogen atom with a positive charge. We call this a hydrogen ion.

There are situations where a hydrogen atom adds extra electrons, but these are rare and of no practical importance here. In physics and in Biohealth, a hydrogen ion is a proton. A hydrogen ion and a proton are the same thing.

What Is pH?

Hydrogen ions determine the composition of fluids in your body. These fluids are either acid or alkaline. Acidity or alkalinity is determined by the amount of hydrogen ions present. The more hydrogen ions present, the more acid the tissue or fluid is. The fewer hydrogen ions present, the more alkaline the tissue or fluid is. Acidity or alkalinity is thus produced by an electrical charge which is the result of the number of the hydrogen ions present.

The amount or degree of acidity or alkalinity is measured by what is called pH. Since acidity-alkalinity is determined by the number of hydrogen ions present, pH is a measure of the hydrogen ions present.

pH stands for "potential hydrogen." Potential hydrogen is a measure of how many more hydrogen ions can be added to a given solution. The more hydrogen ions present, the fewer that can be added. When you have a low pH, fewer hydrogen ions can be added so more hydrogen ions are present. The lower the pH, the more hydrogen ions that are present and the more acid the solution.

pH is ranked by a number from zero to 14. At zero pH, no more hydrogen ions can be added and the fluid is as acid as possible. At a pH of 14, the maximum number of hydrogen ions can be added and the tissue is as alkaline as possible. A pH of 7 is neutral and is neither acid nor alkaline.

The lower the pH is below 7.0, the more hydrogen ions are present. Hydrogen ions are positively charged so the more hydrogen ions that are present, the greater the positive charge and the greater the acidity in the fluid. The higher the pH number is above 7.0, the fewer the number of hydrogen ions present and the less the positive charge and more alkaline the fluid is.

Now, here's the payoff: pH has great significance to health. The more acid an organ or tissue is, the greater the number of hydrogen ions present, the greater the positive electrical charge, and the more activity and strength in the organ or tissue.

The more alkaline an organ or tissue is, the fewer hydrogen ions present, the lower the positive electrical charge, and the less activity and strength the alkaline organ or tissue will have.

All this fits in well with the information presented in the last chapter on magnetism. pH goes beyond just acidity and alkalinity to the creation of magnetic fields and the resulting physical and behavioral effects we discussed. A low pH, which indicates an excess of hydrogen ions, is associated with a south pole magnetic field. A high pH, which indicates a low number of hydrogen ions, is associated with a north pole magnetic field. As outlined in the last chapter, the effects of polar opposites are significant and of huge importance to the Biohealth System.

What Is Functional Energy? Functional Health?

Each part of your body requires the correct energy for it to function correctly. *Correct functional energy* is the energy level at which an organ or body part does its job the best. Correct functional energy produces functional health.

Correct functional energy, and the functional health it produces, is a matter of hydrogen ions. If there is an excess of hydrogen ions (too acid) or a deficiency of hydrogen ions (too alkaline), the bioenergy of the organ or tissue is out of balance and it cannot do its job properly.

Functional health is thus a measure of hydrogen ions. There is a correct number of hydrogen ions for every organ, gland, or tissue in the body. When that number is somehow changed, ineffective and incorrect function results. The correct number of hydrogen ions produces balanced bioenergy. Balanced bioenergy produces correct function which is functional health. Thus, your body functions correctly only when it has the correct number of hydrogen ions. Hydrogen ions define functional energy and functional health.

Functional pH and Balancing Bioenergy

When we talk about functional energy and say an area or organ is too acid or alkaline, we are not talking about actual pH, or the pH we talked about above. We are talking about *functional pH*.

Functional pH is the pH that produces balanced bioenergy and functional health in a specific body part or organ. It is the pH at which the organ or body part does its job the best. This varies widely from the actual pH numbers listed previously. Each organ and tissue in your body has its own functional pH.

Functional pH varies for different parts of the body. For instance, in your stomach a pH of 1 is normal. In your blood, a pH of 1 would indicate death. If you look into a physiology textbook, you'll see a list of widely differing functional pH numbers for each organ in your body.

Functional pH also varies widely depending on situation and the individual involved. That's why your testing magnet is so important. It tells you if an organ is functioning with too much acid (too many hydrogen ions) or too much alkaline (too few) for the conditions and stress level under which you're living. The testing magnet measures your condition at the moment and is always immediately relevant.

The correct number of hydrogen ions, correct pH and correct bioenergy are all, basically, one entity. When you have one, you have them all, and when they are correct, your body produces health. You have a balanced bioenergy field.

As you know, a balanced bioenergy field produces healthy organs and a healthy body. Imbalanced bioenergy fields produce malfunctioning organs and disease, and hydrogen ions play a major role in each. In the next chapter we'll talk more about hydrogen ions and their link to imbalanced bioenergy and disease.

CHAPTER 8

How Cellular Change Leads to Malfunction and Disease

Throw up the windows, open wide the doors, let generosity, let the high purpose of happiness be the dominating impulse in every situation that confronts us.

—Llewelyn Powys, *Impassioned Clay*

Let's take a look at the origin and nature of disease from a Biohealth perspective, which is quite different from that of modern medicine. The medical system is still, basically, in the "disease" business. It focuses on disease and illness, which often allows the health problems to remain.

Biohealth is in the "wellness" business. Our focus is on health. Disease is not the enemy in the Biohealth System. We don't obsess on it or use it as a catalyst for depression. Disease provides us with an opportunity to further our knowledge about ourselves and all that is around us. It is a condition that provides us a chance to learn more about the way our body works.

It is, in a way, a classroom for better living. It can be an experience that will ultimately bring you to a much greater knowingness of health. Our goal is for you to learn how to get your body to produce health. Once we've created the environment of health in your body, disease is no longer an issue.

Disease and Reversed Polarity

Your body is made up of cells. They are the building blocks for function and life. When you have healthy cells you have a healthy body and healthy life. When you have diseased cells, you have diseased organs and a diseased body.

Each cell in your body has two major parts: the nucleus and the cytoplasm. The nucleus is the "center" of the cell and contains the chromosomes, DNA and other material responsible for directing the activity of the cell. The cytoplasm makes up the body of the cell and contains the cell's working parts, which are called *organelles*.

Each cell in your body produces life energy for your body. As an automobile runs on gasoline, your body runs on life energy. In a healthy cell the nucleus of the cell is electropositive and the cytoplasm is electronegative. The nucleus spins clockwise and the cytoplasm spins counterclockwise. This produces life energy, the bioenergy your body needs for health.

In disease, the polarity and spin of the cell are reversed. The nucleus becomes electronegative. The cytoplasm becomes electropositive. The nucleus spins counterclockwise. The cytoplasm spins clockwise. Everything is reversed from what it was in the healthy cell. As a result, the cell no longer produces enough energy. Disease begins when the cells of an organ reverse polarity, reverse their spin and stop producing sufficient energy.

The Two Major Stages of Cell Disease

There are two major stages to the disease process in a cell. In the first, reverse polarity occurs. Cells become too weak to produce enough bioenergy to function correctly. The cells and the organs they make up simply do not have enough bioenergy to do their job.

The reason this occurs is that the cells do not have enough hydrogen ions and are too alkaline for healthy function. They will test as north pole with our testing magnet (in Chapter 10 you will do north and south pole testing) and this imbalance has a severe effect on cellular activity.

In stage two, the body tries to strengthen the weak cell by sending much-needed hydrogen ions into it but this doesn't work because whatever prevented the cell from functioning correctly in the first place has not been corrected. Instead of restoring proper function the hydrogen ions produce a stronger malfunctioning cell.

The malfunctioning cells need more than an influx of hydrogen ions to return to health. They need to correct the cause of the reversed polarity. Unfortunately, as the hydrogen ions continue to flood in, they actually worsen the situation. What evolves is a strong diseased cell. Since it has an excess of hydrogen ions, it is positive and will give a south pole test magnet reading. The stage two diseased cell is much more difficult to correct than a stage one cell.

The stage one north pole diseased cell is weak and does not produce enough energy. Being weak, however, it does not take much energy from the body. The stage two south pole diseased cell is very strong because it has many hydrogen ions. It not only does not produce energy for the body, but it robs hydrogen ions from the body and it robs a great deal of energy from the entire body. Thus the stage two diseased cell is a double dose of trouble. It delivers a two-punch combination to the cell that can ultimately lead to a knockout.

A vicious circle begins. The more hydrogen ions that come to the south pole diseased cells, the more unbalanced the bioenergy becomes. The more unbalanced the cell's bioenergy becomes, the more hydrogen ions come into it and the stronger it becomes. The more diseased it becomes, the stronger it becomes and the more energy it takes from the body.

This is why bacterial infections and cancer are so dangerous and often fatal. Cancer cells become so strong and take so much energy from the rest of the body so quickly that the deterioration of health is often stunning in its speed and extent.

My former mentor and partner, Dr. Richard Broeringmeyer, did extensive research in this area. He found that when stage two cells take away 35 percent of the energy of the body, the heart stops beating. He also found that when stage two cells take away 30 percent of the energy of the body, it is very often impossible to restore health.

Why Do Cells Become Diseased?

There are six major reasons why cells reverse polarity and become diseased:

1. Incorrect nutrition

2. Stress

3. Toxicity

4. Structural problems

5. Lack of proper exercise

6. Incorrect structure

These will be discussed later. The point I'd like to make right now is that, whatever combination of these six caused the cell to become diseased, they must be corrected before the cell can balance its bioenergy and return to health. Unless the causes of disease are corrected, the fertile field that produced the disease will remain. For instance, if stress, toxicity and incorrect nutrition originally caused the disease, each of these must be corrected for the disease to fully disappear.

How You Can Know the Causes of the Disease Have Been Removed

By doing your Biohealth proving with the test magnet you will know when the causes have been removed. When your body, with no help from you or anyone or anything else, restores an energy imbalance to a balance you know the causes are no longer active. Thus, proving is essential to the Biohealth System because proving tells you that the causes of the disease have been removed. At the end of Chapter 12 you will do a proving.

Don't Procrastinate

Time is also of importance here. The sooner in the disease process you begin to correct the problem, the easier it is to correct. In short, a stage one diseased cell is easier to correct than a stage two diseased cell. This is one reason why the Biohealth System stresses continual monitoring and testing of your body. A major goal of the system is to restore balanced energy to the weakened, diseased cells before they become strong, diseased cells.

The earlier in any disease process you start the Biohealth System, the easier and faster you can regain health and the more certain you will succeed. With severe illness, such as cancer and heart disease, we recommend that you start immediately. Indeed, any disease you are now experiencing, whether mild or severe, is your own body telling you to begin your Biohealth Program now.

Every human being has only a limited number of years to live. Any year you waste being sick is forever lost. Likewise, if you want to get older without the pain of aging, if you want to make yourself virtually immune to the diseases called aging, if you want to get control of your own health, you owe it to yourself to start the Biohealth System today.

The Biohealth System will help keep your vitality and zest flowing. It will build immunity to disease. The sooner you begin, the sooner you will be able to live life with the joy and vigor brought by proper function and good health.

The longer you delay achieving good health, the longer you will experience pain, fatigue and the misery of disease. So, how can you possibly wait? The time to start the Biohealth System is immediately.

CHAPTER 9

The Biohealth Personality

No problem can be solved from the same consciousness that created it.

—Albert Einstein

What kind of person does it take to succeed in the Biohealth System?

I'd like to be able to delude myself and say that the Biohealth System is for everybody. I know what the Biohealth System can do and what it can mean. I'd like to believe that everybody, regardless of their personality or commitment, could receive its benefits. But while I know that the Biohealth System can help everyone, I know that some people just aren't ready for it.

Are you ready for the Biohealth System?

To answer this question, I've identified five personal characteristics shared by people who have used the Biohealth System to gain biological health. If you can answer "yes" to each of the questions in this chapter, you're ready to do the step-by-step Biohealth System program that begins in the next chapter.

Question 1
Do You Want to Take Responsibility for Your Own Life?

There are many people who don't take responsibility well. They're frightened by freedom. As long as they're in a conventional authoritarian situation where they're told what to do by others, they're okay. But put them in a comparatively unstructured or free situation and they flounder.

When asked to fall back on their own resources, they find they don't know how. They mistrust their abilities and intellect. Some will become anxious, distrustful or depressed. Without someone to take them by the hand, they're lost. They are overwhelmed by freedom.

People who find responsibility and freedom frightening will be uncomfortable with the Biohealth System. Biohealth is designed around the fact that health is derived internally. To achieve health we communicate with our inner self. No doctor can do this for us. We must do this ourselves!

As a result, if you can't take responsibility for your health Biohealth is not for you. If you believe health comes only from outside your body, Biohealth is not for you.

Question 2
Do You Want to Empower Yourself?

Most health programs and professionals ask you to have faith and believe in them. They want you to put yourself in their hands and have them find the answers for you. In effect, you become their slave. You have to do what they say. They, after all, know what they're doing. You don't.

You become passive in this situation. It's like watching a TV show. You have no control over what happens. You're just another passive viewer of the drama taking place on the picture tube.

By placing our future entirely into the hands of another, we breed uncertainty. We lose control and feel like we're totally at the mercy of forces outside ourselves. We feel threatened. At risk. A prisoner with our fate to be decided by a jury we will have absolutely no influence over. A malfunctioning body also tends to take you prisoner. When you are ill, you become a prisoner of your body. Your body produces constraints. You lose freedom. The extent of your illness limits those things you can and can't do. Disease comes to define your life.

Even if we're "cured" we still live in fear of future disease. Indeed, the fear never seems to end. We're always worried about the next disease lurking around the corner.

When you take control of your own health with the Biohealth System you become empowered. Uncertainty is replaced with knowledge and confidence. Fear is replaced with understanding and with immunity from disease.

As you empower yourself you begin to develop your faculties and abilities. Every time you use the Biohealth System, you open a new door to a different world. It's a world much larger than the one you lived in before you opened your new door, and it is a world with more potential and awareness.

You don't have to live in fear. You can live in knowledge, an ever growing knowledge that will not only make you healthy, but also make you a more effective, stronger human being.

Of course, some people do not want to be empowered. There is responsibility with empowerment. If you don't want to be empowered, if you don't want to take control of your health, the Biohealth System isn't for you.

Question 3
Do You Want to Learn How Your Own Body Works?

Modern therapy lost access to the life forces within our body that produce health. Biohealth seeks to reconnect us with these forces. Biohealth demands that you gain as much information and knowledge about the workings of your bioenergy self as possible. It opens you up to the universe within. In fact, Biohealth is the biggest classroom you'll ever find. It's also a classroom where the learning never ends.

To succeed in the Biohealth System you must have a basic curiosity about yourself. You must be willing to do those things necessary to complete the Biohealth Program. You must be aware and open to your energy body and continue to learn from it.

If you want somebody else to do it all for you, if you want to remain ignorant to the sources of your health, if you want nothing to do with your inner self, the Biohealth System isn't for you.

Question 4
Are You a Person Who Doesn't Look for Excuses?

Everyone I've ever known who was sick looked for excuses for their illness.

"The water isn't purified properly."

"There are too many pesticides in my fruit."

"People keep giving me *their* bugs"

"I'm living under high voltage wires."

"It's the pollution."

And on and on and on and on.

These people are always looking outside their own body for the answer. One of the things I have always focused on in my workshops is that your job in Biohealth is not to create an un-polluted, squeaky clean environment. You're never going to be able to do that. Nor would you want to live in such a sterile, unreal world.

Your job is to create a body that is healthy and immune to disease. Remember that health and disease can't exist in the same body at the same time. Biohealth is more concerned with achieving health and building immunity to disease than building a new world.

Not that we don't want to end pollution, but we don't blame outside forces. Our aim is to build our inner strength. Our concerns are internal. Not external.

106

Biohealth is defined by action. If you're always looking outside yourself for a cause, that's not action. That's paralysis. By being passive and focusing on the world outside yourself you've doomed yourself to inaction.

Biohealth's goal is to create something stronger inside of you than that which is outside, so that your inner forces are superior in strength to those forces outside of you. That's action. And while taking action you also increase your awareness and experience. In fact, through the action you take in the Biohealth System you awaken to a part of your life you'd never been conscious of before.

The Biohealth System is for doers. It revolves around action. If you're an excuse maker, it isn't for you.

Question 5
Can You See Past the Media/Cultural Pitches?

We are a society shaped greatly by television and advertising. From our earliest days, we have been told what we should do.

"Quick as a wink, you're in the pink," says a commercial voice.

A cranky senior citizen takes a headache tablet and *voilà*, he suddenly turns into Grandfather of the Year.

A terminally ill patient goes to a hospital and magically, within the space of an hour he is healed by Super Doctor.

We're taught that if you buy the right product or service or find just the right person, they will all quickly and painlessly solve your troubles for you. In the average advertisement, a person goes from troubled to joyously carefree in the space of 30 seconds, simply because they were willing to spend some bucks on the advertiser's product or service.

Meanwhile, vicariously, we all become characters in an action-adventure show or become the subjects of the nightly news. Sure, that's not us up there on the screen but it just as well might be. We see ourselves and our society in those colorful shadows on the TV screen.

This is important because the world of television is a scary one. There's always some dangerous situation or condition waiting around the next turn to snap us up. And generally, we're not going to be strong enough to provide for our own defense. We've got to buy what the people on the tube are selling us to save ourselves.

When it comes to health care, disease is seen as the "enemy" in our marketing-driven culture. It is to be feared. It is an ever present danger. Indeed, it is often placed in a war-like or battle scenario. We are attacked by nefarious diseases. Death is imminent. All is lost. Then, quite suddenly and heroically, the white knight of modern medicine appears on the field of battle to slay the evil enemy and save the day. Everyone lives happily ever after.

We are taught by health professionals and our media and culture that our health depends on them, the white knights, and not on our own body. We are told we must turn to health professionals to achieve health. That only they have the answers and to be healthy, we must subvert ourselves entirely to their authority and expertise.

Biohealth rejects this view. Freedom from disease doesn't come from any fight or battle. It comes from living in a properly functioning body. It stresses immunity from disease. Its goal is not to fight disease but to create a body in which disease cannot exist.

Disease itself is not seen so much as the "enemy" as it is a learning experience. Disease is an opportunity and challenge to remedy what is wrong, and by so doing move to continually higher levels of health.

If we are to truly achieve health and immunity from disease, if we are to truly grow as individuals and meet our highest potential, we must break out of the disease industry prison our culture and media have created. At the same time, we must reestablish our partnership with our own body.

In applying the Biohealth System we interact with our entire human self, both the outer physical self and our inner life-giving self. Modern medicine prevents us from knowing that innermost self. It separates us from ourselves. Biohealth reestablishes this relationship.

Health Is Something You Do

If you answered "yes" to each of the five previous questions, you're ready for the Biohealth System. If you want to take responsibility for your life and health, empower yourself and learn about the wonderful world within you, Biohealth is for you.

Ultimately, health is not something you have. It is not the result of any diploma on a wall, or testimonials to what is being sold to you. It is not something somebody gives to you.

Health is something you do. It comes with the greatest credential of all, your own body. It is a gift to you from your inner self.

Books, like this one, are all well and good. You can learn a great deal about things by reading books and taking workshops and classes. But the only way you can have knowingness about anything is to directly experience it. And you can only experience what you do.

The Biohealth System is built on the direct experience that results in true knowingness. In the next chapter, you will learn how to produce health.

CHAPTER 10

Creating Health That Lasts—How to Use Magnetic Testing to Achieve Energy Balance

Nothing is more villainous than the way people
of conventional habits endeavor to tame,
correct, and inhibit the wild pleasure of lust.

—Llewelyn Powys, *Glory of Life*

The next four chapters are interactive and will guide you through the Biohealth System. Although we provide you with a written guide here, the key to learning about Biohealth isn't reading. It is doing. Only by doing can you achieve knowingness. Only by doing can you learn the Biohealth System.

At this point in the book, you have a decision to make. If you've skipped to this page from the beginning of the book, we invite you to read on and become more acquainted with the mechanics of the Biohealth System. If you've read through the previous chapters but have not yet decided, read through the remaining chapters to decide if you really want to commit to Biohealth.

But if you've reached this point in the book and are genuinely excited or you have a severe health problem that needs attention, I urge you to order the test and correcting magnets from the company listed in the back of this book immediately. That way you can start performing the procedures you read about right now.

Reading the text is fine. Reading has its place. But only when you directly experience Biohealth by doing it will you know what you can accomplish.

Review

Let's start with a review of the seven steps in the Biohealth Program identified earlier in the book. As you recall, the Biohealth Systems consists of:

1. Testing
2. Restoring bioenergy balance
3. Stopping the autoimmune attack
4. Determining the correct nutrition for you
5. Applying and monitoring the Biohealth Program
6. Proving the program
7. Maintaining correct function

In all but one of these steps you will make use of one or both of the Biohealth magnets. The first magnet you will use is the "test magnet." With this magnet you determine the bioenergetic condition of any organ, gland or tissue in your body. In the Biohealth System it is used both to determine the health of an organ, gland or tissue and to test the effects that different foods, nutritional supplements or other substances will have on the part of the body being tested.

The evaluation done by the test magnet is not quantitative. You won't get numbers like you get with many medical tests. The magnet is a qualitative instrument. It will tell you if the organ being tested is balanced and healthy. It will tell you if it has excessive hydrogen ions and is too acid for correct function or if it has a deficiency of hydrogen ions and is too alkaline for correct function.

It does not tell you how much of an excess or deficiency the organ has. It doesn't have to. Whatever the extent of the excess or deficiency, the System will work to correct it until balance has been achieved.

The second type of magnet is the "correcting magnet." This magnet is used to correct the bioenergy imbalance of the organ tested.

Both magnets are essential to the Biohealth System. The "correcting magnet" is used in step 2. It plays a primary role in restoring bioenergy balance to the body. The "test magnet" is used in steps 1, 4, 5, 6 and 7. It is your tool for determining what the body needs for health and when your body is healthy.

The Testing Magnet

The test magnet is not as simple as it looks. It took a great deal of time, effort and knowledge to design it. It had to be constructed with three requirements in mind:

1. Separation between north and south poles

2. Creation of the correct amount of energy to ensure an accurate reading

3. Proper sizing so the part of the body being tested—and only that part—will respond

The first requirement involved the need for a magnet that allowed reliable testing with either a north or south pole. In our chapter on magnets, we discussed how opposite poles attract each other. To keep the energy of each pole as pure north and south as they can be, the two poles must somehow be sepa-

South Pole

Test magnet - actual size

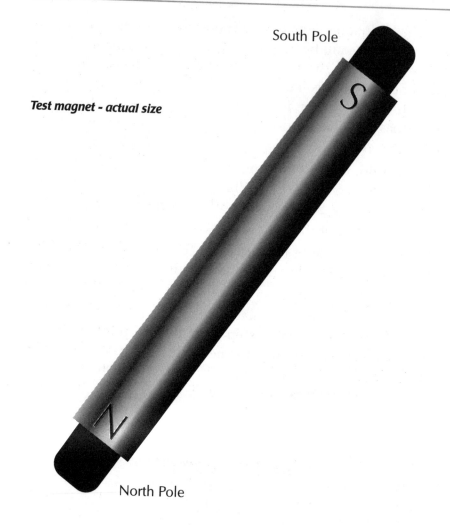

North Pole

rated. This was done with a steel casing placed in the test magnet between the two poles.

A magnet is more strongly attracted to steel than to another magnetic field. By putting a collar of steel between the two poles, the steel attracts magnetic energy before it gets to the other pole. With most of the energy attracted to the steel, very little gets to the other pole to affect its field. In this way, north and south poles are isolated from each other. When you test with them, you will see the effects of a single pole and not a combination of fields.

The second requirement for the testing magnet is two requirements. First, it has to properly stress the organ being tested. You will learn later in this chapter that Biohealth tests the health of an organ by testing its response to stress. Second, it has to have the correct strength to stress the organ being tested. The optimum strength of the test magnet was determined to be 1,000 gauss. This is the correct gauss for testing because it penetrates to the organ, gland or tissue to be tested without affecting the area around or beyond it.

If the test magnet was too weak, it wouldn't penetrate to the proper level or test the entire area. If it was too strong, it would test too large an area or penetrate too deeply and test more than the organ being tested. As built, the test magnet is not a random magnet but one specifically designed to affect the proper area with just enough stress to get an accurate response and result.

The third requirement for the test magnet is proper size. If you put too large a magnet on, you'd have no idea whether you were testing the target organ or an area much larger. Likewise, a smaller magnet could cause problems in the other direction. The testing magnet we use is just the right size for stressing only the organs, glands and tissues targeted by the Biohealth System.

The Test Magnet

When you test an organ with the test magnet, you read the results by the effect it has on muscles. You can test either arm muscles or the muscles in the legs.

Testing the arm is by far the most popular and widely used method. It is the most convenient and easy to do. Testing on the knee, when it can be done, is also very simple. The leg length test is harder to learn and perform but is very accurate. We will discuss all three but will first concentrate on the arm.

The arm test is very simple. After applying the test magnet to the organ being tested, you simply check the arm for weakness (we'll talk about how to do this in a moment). If the arm goes weak, that means the organ is positive.

Positive means there is a bioenergy imbalance in the organ. When you test the south pole and the arm goes weak, the organ has an excess of hydrogen ions and is too acid to function correctly. It is a positive test for an excess of hydrogen ions. The organ is said to be "south pole."

When you test with the north pole and the arm goes weak, that organ has a deficiency of hydrogen ions and is too alkaline to function correctly. It is a positive test for a deficiency of hydrogen ions. The organ is said to be "north pole."

Tests on the knee and legs are similar in nature. If the knee weakens, the test is positive in the same way as the arm test above. If heels move so leg length changes occur in the leg length test (also called the "body distortion test") the test is also positive. Results are very reliable.

But why do we get a "positive" result, and why do these tests work so well?

The Emergency Muscle Reaction—How Your Body Tells You Something Is Wrong

Whenever an emergency occurs in your body, you get a reflex reaction to get away from whatever is causing the emergency. Under normal circumstances, information is received through your sensory nerves, transmitted to your central nervous system (CNS) and from there, to your brain. The brain then decides how to respond and sends this information back to your CNS. The CNS transmits this information to your motor nerves and you ultimately end up taking the actions your brain decided you should take.

However, in an emergency, you do not have this kind of time. An instant response—as instant a response as possible—is needed. A common example of this involves laying your hand on a hot surface, like a stove. You do not have time to ask your brain what to do. By the time it came up with a response, your hand could be badly burned.

That's why, in an emergency situation, you get a reflex action where information is short circuited. Information does not go from your sensory nerves to the brain. It goes only to the CNS from where a message is rapidly sent to your muscles to immediately do something to get you away from whatever is causing the emergency. This short circuit is called a *reflex*, which occurs whenever the body gets an emergency message. An emergency message says harm may occur unless immediate action is taken. This is exactly what happens when you use the test magnet. You are creating a reflex response from the organ being tested.

This is one of the great things about the test magnet. It has been designed to affect only a specific organ or body part and to give a reflex response. Using just any magnet will not do this. Only a correctly designed test magnet will give us the single organ reflex response we desire.

How the Test Magnet Creates an Emergency Response

Assume, for a moment, you have an organ that is out of balance because it has too many hydrogen ions and is too acid. When south pole energy is put into that organ by placing the south pole of your test magnet over it, it increases an already excessive and harmful hydrogen ion concentration.

Increasing an already excessive hydrogen ion concentration is an emergency. This increase can do harm to your body, and knowing this, your body gives you an emergency muscle reaction. A reflex reaction. The body says, "Stop! Don't do this!" Your muscles go weak.

If muscles go weak when the south pole is applied, your body is telling you the organ being tested is out of balance and has an excess of hydrogen ions. If muscles go weak when the north pole is applied, your body is telling you the organ being tested is out of balance and has a deficiency of hydrogen ions.

117

As described previously, most people choose the arm muscles (actually the deltoid muscle at the top of the arm) to test. After the arm has shown weakness to the application of one pole of the magnet, it will show strength when the other pole is applied. Why does the arm become strong with the other pole?

Arm weakness (called a "positive" response) tells you that you are increasing an existing imbalance. When the arm subsequently goes strong with the opposite pole, it is telling you that the opposite pole is correcting the existing imbalance. Indeed, the arm going strong on the opposite pole confirms your original reading.

When the south pole produces arm weakness and the north pole produces arm strength, it verifies the reading that an excess of hydrogen ions is present. The south pole of the test magnet makes the situation worse. The north improves it. The opposite is also true. When the north pole produces arm weakness and the south pole produces arm strength, this confirms that not enough hydrogen ions are present. The south pole adds needed hydrogen ions while the north pole only makes the deficiency worse.

This is an important principle. When you apply the opposite pole to the one that tested positive, it helps correct the bioenergy imbalance in the organ. That's why, with the correcting magnet, we use the pole opposite to what gave the positive response. We'll discuss this further in the next chapter.

What Is Balanced Bioenergy?

Now hear this! You are not testing for specific levels of acidity or alkalinity when you use a test magnet. Sure, there are many tests out there that will claim to give you a right or wrong pH for organs, but we haven't found them to be very accurate. This is because the acidity or alkalinity of an organ or tissue *changes* depending on the stress under which it is functioning.

The health of an organ isn't measurable by a standard pH reading. It's normal for an organ to go acid or alkaline in response to stress. pH levels can vary widely and still be indicative of nothing more than the day-to-day stresses of living.

Likewise, balanced bioenergy is not a constant, unchanging condition. What balanced bioenergy means is that the organ can go out of balance in response to stress and then return itself to balanced bioenergy. It is its return to balanced bioenergy that tells you an organ is healthy.

Health is never static but is dynamic. Unbalanced bioenergy and disease exist in an organ that responds to stress but cannot return to balance. If an organ responds to stress and returns to balance, it has health.

This brings us to another important point about the design of the test magnet. The test magnet produces exactly the amount of stress necessary to properly test the ability of an organ to respond to that stress and return to normal. The organ is neither overstressed nor understressed. The magnet provides just enough stress to properly test the organ and nothing more. When an organ has the ability to respond to the stress of the south pole of the test magnet and return to balance, and respond to the north pole of the test magnet and return to balance with no resulting emergency response from the body and no arm weakness on either pole, the organ being tested has bioenergy balance and is healthy.

Placing the Test Magnet Over the Area to Be Tested

Test Magnet Placement— How to Test Bioenergy Balance in Your Body

To test an organ or tissue, place the test magnet directly over it. The magnet can be put directly in contact with the skin or against tight-fitting clothing. Use of the magnet may sometimes irritate the skin and tight-fitting clothing will guard against irritation while keeping the magnet near enough to the organ to be effective.

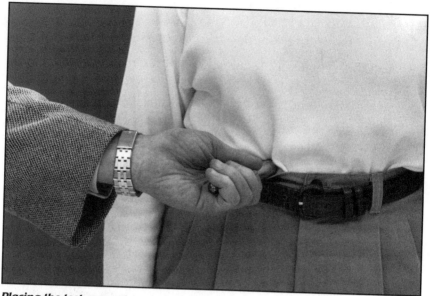

Placing the test magnet.

You can start with either the north or south pole of the magnet over the organ to be tested. Whichever pole you choose, the tip of the magnet should be over the area being evaluated. It doesn't matter if the tip of the tip or the side of the tip is over the organ, just as long as the tip of the magnet is over it. In most cases the magnet is aimed directly at the area being tested.

After testing one pole by observing arm weakness as described below, we apply the other pole and perform the same procedure. It's that simple.

Step-by-Step Procedure for Observing Arm Muscle Weakness

The arm muscle test is done by two people. The first person is the subject being tested. The second is the examiner, the person doing the testing. For the sake of this discussion, we're going to take the position of the examiner as we walk through the process.

First, have the subject stand in a comfortable position. Then have him or her extend an arm, preferably the left arm, straight out to the side.

120

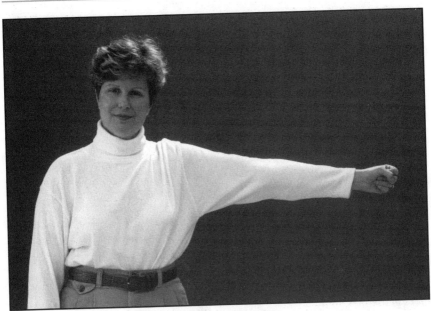

Subject extends arm straight out and makes a fist.

The fingers can also be placed straight out with the palm facing down and the thumb extended forward or held against the hand as shown.

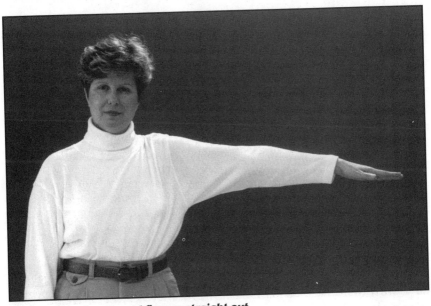

Subject extends arm and fingers straight out.

The palm can also face forward with the fingers held straight out and the thumb extended upwards or against the hand. You can try any of the hand configurations above. Experiment and use the one which works best for your subject.

The fist is usually the stronger configuration, so if you have someone with a weak arm, it is usually the best to use. The weaker position is usually the one with the fingers straight out and thumb extended. For subjects with very strong arms, usually use it. Find the best position for any subject through trial and error.

The examiner now determines the correct "testing pressure." This is very important. To do this he or she presses on the wrist of the subject's extended arm. Press hard enough to get a very slight downward movement on the arm until a slight bounce is felt. This will give you the approximate level of pressure to apply to that subject. This is the "testing pressure."

If you press the wrist of the subject harder or lighter than the testing pressure, you may get a false reading. Learning how to determine the testing pressure is of prime importance. Testing the strength of the subject's arm by pressing on the wrist—when there is a slight give—is the correct strength to use to test the subject.

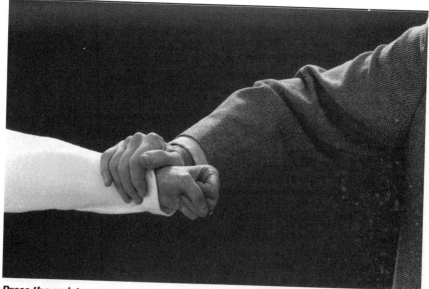

Press the wrist.

Once you've determined the subject's testing pressure, you can place the north or south pole of the test magnet over the organ or tissue to be tested and using the test pressure, test that organ or gland. However, before you test the arm by applying testing pressure to it, tell the subject to resist the pressure. If you apply pressure before the subject resists, the arm will go down every time and you won't get a reliable response. The subject must resist before downward pressure is applied.

With a positive reading indicating an energy imbalance, the arm of the person being tested will go weak. To be dramatic and illustrate the situation to the subject, we will often push the arm down with only one or two fingers.

Then you place the other pole over the organ and test the arm again. If it went weak on the first pole, it will be strong when the opposite pole is applied. This is a very dramatic moment for the subject and convincingly confirms the validity of the test.

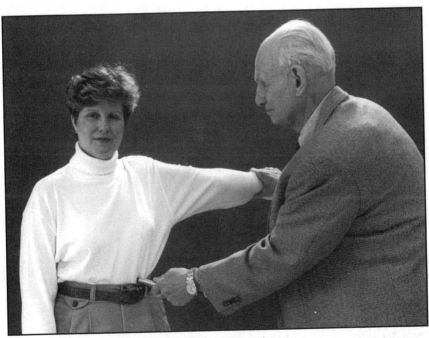

Placing the test magnet and pressing on the wrist.

123

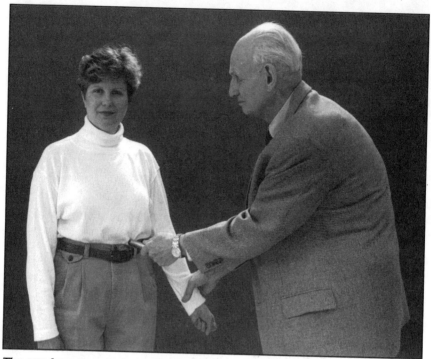

The arm becomes weak and goes down.

To review, if you test the south pole and the arm goes weak, the arm will be strong during the test with the north pole of the magnet because the north pole energy corrects the imbalance. This combination indicates an excess of hydrogen ions in the tissue being tested and a positive south pole imbalance.

The exact opposite occurs with a north pole imbalance. The arm goes weak during the north pole test and strong with the south pole, indicating too few hydrogen ions are present in the tissue.

A Big Advantage

One big advantage Biohealth testing has is that it is not affected by the mind or body of the examiner. In muscle testing done without magnets, outside forces—including the mind and beliefs of the examiner—can give false readings. When the examiner believes an arm should be strong or weak, that belief will often cause the arm to be strong or weak. The test will reflect the belief of the examiner instead of the bioenergy of the subject.

As a result, without the use of magnets, the mind of the examiner must be perfectly neutral because any beliefs or opinions in the mind of the examiner can give a false reading.

Likewise, whenever the examiner touches another person's arm in a nonmagnetic test anything out of balance in the examiner may show up in the person being tested. For instance, if the examiner has a bad liver that bad liver can show up in the analysis being done on the subject. This leaves us with the problem of having to test the tester to make sure they don't have a problem that will show up in the analysis of the test subject.

You don't have to worry about this in the Biohealth System. When testing the arm with magnetic energy we do not get false readings. Magnetic energy is more powerful than the energy the body or mind of the examiner produces. It overcomes it and ensures a reliable measurement.

It's the same with general environmental conditions. Pleasant or unpleasant physical environments can have an effect on muscle testing programs that do not use a magnet, but they do not affect magnetic muscle testing at all.

For example, listening to classical music can balance one's bioenergy just as the correcting magnet does. Thus, listening to classical music during a testing session can give a false balanced reading. Likewise, rock music can unbalance your bioenergy. Listening to rock during a testing session can produce false positive readings. This won't happen when you use the magnet. Even with classical or rock music playing, you will get correct readings.

This is one of the big pluses for magnetic Biohealth testing. With other testing, you have to be concerned that the mind or a physical deficiency of the examiner will show up in the person being examined. The physical environment in which the test takes place may also find its way into the results. Not so with the magnets.

With magnetic testing you know you'll get the result of the magnetic arm test. We know it is the magnetic field that caused her or his arm to go weak. This knowledge is both exciting and empowering.

Surrogate Testing

For the majority of people, arm muscle testing works fine. But for some, the procedure cannot be done. I have tested people who have just had rotator cuff surgery, for instance, and their arm is much too weak to test. The slightest pressure with a single finger would press it down. I have tested women with the same problem. They just couldn't work up any resistance to the arm pressure.

There are other people whose arms are so strong that, even when they go weak, you are not able to push the arm down. Athletes, weight lifters and just about anyone with superior strength in the arm could fit into this category.

In either of these cases, you can use a surrogate for the test. This surrogate can be anybody whose arm is not too strong or weak to perform the test. They serve as a surrogate by substituting their arm for the arm of the test subject and responding for them.

The surrogate procedure begins with the surrogate and test subject interlocking one of their hands with one of the other's. We usually prefer the right hand of the subject interlocking with the left hand of the surrogate. The surrogate then holds his or her other arm straight out while continuing to hold the hand of the person being tested. The test magnet is then applied to the organ of the subject, i.e., the person being tested.

At this point, you push on the surrogate's extended arm as if it were the test subject's. If the surrogate's arm goes down when the south pole of the test magnet is being used, this means the test subject has an excess of hydrogen ions in the tissue being examined. If the surrogate's arm goes down when the north pole is applied to the test subject, there is a north pole imbalance in the subject. If there is no weakness on either pole and the surrogate's arm stays strong, you know the tissue or organ being tested is healthy.

Any energy imbalance in the test subject will be transmitted from the test subject into the surrogate he or she is holding hands with. The surrogate's arm will be weakened by this and when pressure is applied, his or her arm will go down. The surrogate thus registers the reading you would normally get with the test subject were his or her arm not too weak or strong for the test itself.

Knee Testing

The arm muscle test requires two people and some cooperative effort but it is really not difficult. All you need to do is to train the person who will be doing the testing how to push the subject's arm down. In our workshops, we deal mostly with pairs. That way the pair, often a husband and wife, can trade off testing each other.

But there is a way you can become both tester and subject and do your testing solo: knee testing. It's much more difficult to perform than arm testing but some people are able to use it successfully.

To begin, sit comfortably in a good chair, then raise either your left or right leg—whichever you think is weaker—and press firmly against the raised knee. If you can get your knee to give you a little bounce, you will probably be able to do this test. As above, you must experiment a bit to see how much pressure you need to apply to get your knee to go slightly down. That is your testing pressure.

If your leg is so strong that you cannot get it to give you a bounce when you press it, you cannot use this test. You must use the arm, surrogate or leg distortion test, which follows.

If you can get a working test pressure, you can begin the procedure by raising the knee. With one hand, hold your test magnet over the organ you are testing. With the other hand, press on your knee with the correct test pressure. If the leg weakens, it indicates a positive response for that test. Complete the test with the other pole and evaluate results in the same way as with the arm test.

Testing by Observing
Body Distortion (Leg Length)

We can also test for energy imbalance by observing body distortion (changes in leg length). This procedure takes more time and practice to learn. I usually reserve body distortion instruction for an advanced workshop, but if learned properly, it is a reliable tool.

The procedure requires two people. The subject is placed on a table, couch or bed. His or her legs are straightened out. A pillow is placed under the head and the subject is told to relax. (Relaxation is very important here.) Preferably, the subject should be wearing shoes with heels. This is because observing the heels on shoes makes it easier to see leg length changes.

Both heels should be in contact with the table, couch or bed. The toes should be pointed outward, hanging relaxed and looking relaxed. If the toes are pointing straight upward or inward, the subject is not relaxed and the test will not work.

Stand facing the bottom of the feet of your subject. Place your hands under the heel and ankle of each leg. Cup your hands in such a way that the legs lie passively in your hand. With the legs passively in your hands, the heels of each shoe should be exactly even with each other. Both legs should be of the same length.

With the legs held passively in each hand and the subject relaxed, practice picking up the legs so the heels remain even with each other. One leg does not get longer than the other. You must be able to raise both legs without causing one leg to be shorter. With both heels cupped in your hands, lift the feet 8 to 12 inches, then lower them again. During the lifting, keep both heels very close to each other so you can see any changes that occur while you are lifting the feet. You must learn to raise the legs so the heels remain opposite each other with no change in leg length.

The goal here is for the tester to "passively" lift the feet, which means the tester learns to lift the feet without causing any change in leg length during the lifting. When the tester can reliably lift the legs 8 to 12 inches with no change in leg length, he or she is ready to do the testing.

The test begins with a second person placing the test magnet over the organ, gland or tissue to be tested. With the test magnet in place, passively pick up both legs. If the heels move so that one leg becomes shorter than the other, no matter which leg, a body distortion has occurred. This distortion indicates an emergency muscle reaction to the applied magnetic energy.

This is the same situation as when the arm became weak during the arm test. With a change in the position of the heels, you have a positive response to the test magnet. This constitutes a positive reading and indicates an excess or deficiency in hydrogen ions in the tissue being tested.

Complete the test with the other pole and evaluate results as above.

Note: Magnets are not recommended for pregnant women or for people wearing pacemakers or other implanted medical devices.

Learning the basics of using the test magnet is the foundation for the Biohealth System. The test magnet is the first step in our seven-step procedure and it's a primary component of steps 4 to 7. It provides the Biohealth window through which you can "see" your body.

CHAPTER 11

The Basic Magnetic Examination

*The more we overcome our congenital apathy,
our lumpish disposition to take for granted the
deep mystery of existence, the more do we fulfill
the design of being alive.*

—Llewelyn Powys, *Damnable Opinions*

In this chapter you will begin to apply the principles of the Biohealth System. If you have your test magnet in hand, you will directly experience what Biohealth does and realize its potential for your life.

Before you can test, however, you have to know where to test, which is what this chapter is about. In the pages that follow, you will be given a program for testing 22 important places in your body for bioenergy balance and health. The basic magnetic examination is one of a kind—I know of no other examination that gives you anything like it. All 22 sites target major organs, glands and tissues and, with our detailed descriptions, they can all be easily located and tested by following the easy-to-locate landmarks on the body.

Once you become proficient testing these areas, there is no limit to where you can go with the Biohealth System. These 22 areas provide a basic examination of the body but they aren't the only sites available. Muscles, joints—any body tissue or malfunctioning body part—can be tested by the magnet. Indeed, you can test anywhere in your body at any time you feel it should be done.

The test sites are easy to find. For example, suppose you wanted to test your pancreas. Two of the important "body identification markers" on the surface of your body are the nipple lines and the navel (belly button) line. From your left nipple, mentally draw a vertical line straight down your body. Now, from your navel, mentally draw a horizontal line extending across the left side of your body.

The point where these two lines meet, the vertical left nipple line and the horizontal left navel line, is directly above the pancreas. To magnetically test the pancreas you place the test magnet where the two lines intersect. What could be simpler?

The Basic Examination

The 22 areas tested in the basic examination are:

1. Pancreas
2. Liver
3. Gall bladder
4. Adrenal glands
5. Kidneys
6. Thyroid gland
7. Parathyroid glands
8. Stomach
9. Hiatal hernia test
10. Thymus gland
11. Spleen
12. Uterus
13. Ovaries
14. Prostate gland
15. Urinary bladder
16. Colon
17. Diverticulitis test
18. Pituitary gland
19. Pineal gland
20. Heart
21. Lungs
22. Blood

All of these organs and test sites are easily located by using body identification markers:

1. On the surface of your body (surface identification markers)
2. Bones (bone identification markers)
3. Muscles (muscle identification markers)

As you read the following descriptions of where these markers are, I urge you to look at the illustrations provided and locate the markers on your own body as you go.

Identification Markers on the Surface of Your Body

1. The right and left nipple lines. These are vertical lines mentally drawn from you nipples straight downward.
2. The midline is a vertical line down the middle of the body.
3. The navel or belly button line. This is a horizontal line drawn through the belly button.
4. The hipbone line, visualized from the top of the hip bone on one side to the top of the hip bone on the other side.
5. The clavicle (shoulder bone) line.

Identification Markers on the Surface of Your Body

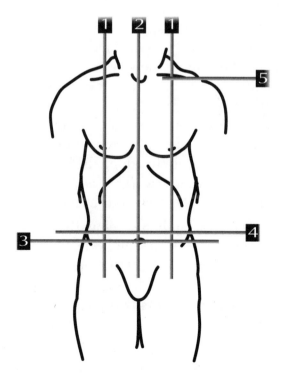

Bone Identification Markers

Bone identification markers are found by locating specific bones of the body. Five major bone markers are used in the Biohealth System. They are described below. Take the time to find them on the diagram below and locate them on your own body as directed. Since you are locating bones, don't be afraid to press firmly on them.

1. The sternum, otherwise known as the breastbone. Run your finger down the front of your neck. It will fall into a notch at the top of a bone. That bone is the sternum. Run your finger down from the notch, which is the top of the sternum, to the bottom of the bone. You will feel a soft spot there. The bone between the notch at the top of your neck and the soft spot at the bottom is the sternum.

2. The clavicle, or shoulder bone. It is the horizontal bone that runs from the top of your sternum over to your shoulder. From the top of your sternum, run your finger along the bone that extends out to your shoulder on each side. This is your clavicle.

3. The ribs. The ribs are shaped in an arc and go downwards and sideways from the sternum. Find your bottom rib, which begins at the bottom of the sternum, and follow it downward and sideways all the way around to the side of your body. That is the bottom of your lowest anterior (front) rib. Next, on the side of your back, go slightly lower than where the anterior rib was, push in and come up until you feel the bottom of the lowest rib. Touching the bottom of the lowest rib, follow it up and inward. That is your lowest "floating" back rib and it is attached to your backbone.

4. Top of the pelvis or hip bone. Below the bottom ribs, press your fingers into the side of your body. They will go in. Now move downward until you feel the top of a bone. That is the top of your hip bone. Find the top of the hip bone on each side of the body and mentally draw a line between them. That is your hip bone line.

Bone Identification Markers

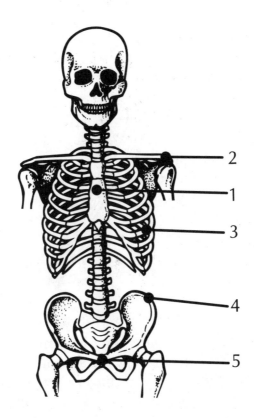

5. The pubic symphysis. The pubic symphysis is a fibrocartilage joint between the left and right hip bones. To find it, run the flat of your hand down your midline from your belly button until you hit a bone. This is the top of your hip bone where the two sides join. It is the top of the pubic symphysis.

Muscle Identification Markers

Sternocleidomastoid Muscle (SCM) and Right Carotid Artery

We will only need to identify one muscle, the sternocleidomastoid muscle in the side of the neck. We will also need to identify the nearby carotid artery.

Sternocleidomastoid Muscle (SCM) and Right Carotid Artery

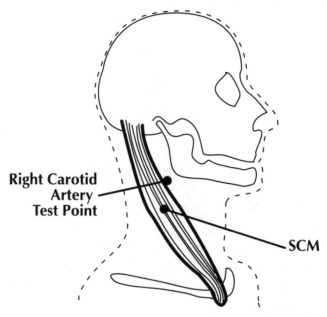

**Right Carotid
Artery
Test Point**

SCM

The sternocleidomastoid muscle. This muscle is in the side of your neck. It feels like a rope. To find it, feel underneath the point of your chin. Slide your finger along the jawbone toward your ear and the side of your neck. You will feel the jawbone curve up. Beyond this point, on your neck, you can feel something like a rope. Grab it between your thumb and fingers and follow it down your neck. The muscle will go forward and downward ending at the level of the clavicle close to your midline. You have now identified your sternocleidomastoid muscle.

The right carotid artery. Just in front the sternocleidomastoid muscle on the right side of your neck is the right carotid artery. Midway down your neck, feel for a pulse or heartbeat just in front of the muscle. When you've found it, you've found the carotid artery.

Follow the carotid artery up (along the front of the SCM muscle) until you get to the back of the mandible where it starts to turn up. You will feel heartbeat in this area. This is the area of the carotid bifurcation, and this will be your test point for the blood.

Where and How to Test

The following material will give a detailed description, with illustrations, of where to test for the 22 different organs, glands or tissues in the basic examination. We'll be using body identification markers to find each of the 22 test areas. First, you will get a short overview on the nature of the organ or test area itself and then a written description of how to find it. At the end of the chapter are several diagrams giving you a visual perspective of where each test point is. You should be able to do Biohealth testing when you complete this chapter.

1. Pancreas

The glands in your body fall into two main groups—exocrine and endocrine. Exocrine glands secrete their products into ducts, or channels, that carry them to the outside of the body or body cavities. The salivary and sweat glands are both exocrine glands.

Endocrine glands produce hormones and empty them directly into the bloodstream.

There is one gland in the body that performs both exocrine and endocrine functions—the pancreas.

The pancreas is, functionally, two organs in one. Most of the pancreas is an exocrine gland that produces digestive enzymes which are carried by ducts to the intestines where they break down food and promote digestion. As an endocrine gland, the pancreas produces two important hormones—insulin and glucagon—that regulate the metabolism of the carbohydrates we eat. Inadequate secretion of insulin by the pancreas can cause a severe form of the disease diabetes mellitus.

The pancreas is very easy to find. It is located at the intersection of the vertical left nipple line and the horizontal navel or belly button line.

2. The Liver

The liver is the largest gland in the body, weighing between 3 and 5 pounds. It is a workhorse organ, performing more than 500 known functions.

Food that has gone through the digestive system, as well as toxins of intestinal origin, must pass through the liver. Inappropriate materials like bacteria, insoluble materials, drugs and hormones are removed from the blood in the liver and materials needed by the body are put into general circulation in the liver. The liver also breaks down fats and proteins and stores vitamins such as A, B_{12}, D, E and K and minerals such as iron and copper.

One of the most important functions of the liver is the production of bile. Bile helps the body digest and absorb fatty foods and get rid of waste products. The liver is the major area in the body where detoxification takes place.

The liver is located on the right nipple line down the front of your body. It begins just above the lowest (twelfth rib) and extends upward to about the ninth rib. We prefer to test on the nipple line between the lowest two ribs.

3. Gall Bladder

The gall bladder stores and concentrates bile until it is needed in the digestive process. To find the gall bladder, go down to the bottom of the lowest rib on your right side and move your fingers along the bottom of the rib from the right side of your body towards the middle. You will find what feels like a corner on the rib. This is the common bile duct. This is where you measure both the common bile duct and the gall bladder.

4. Adrenal Glands

There are two adrenal glands and two major components of each gland. The outer tissue of the adrenal gland is called the cortex and the inner tissue is called the medulla.

One hormone from the cortex regulates the body's concentration of electrolytes, a solution that conducts electricity in the body. Another helps metabolize carbohydrates, proteins and fats. Others serve as anti-inflammatories and produce sex hormones which supplement the sex hormones from the gonads.

The medulla produces a series of hormones that prepare the body for muscular action and greater physical performance. Stress has a large effect on the adrenals and can cause the glands to secrete 20 times the usual amount of these hormones.

Overall, the adrenal glands secrete more than three dozen hormones and play an essential role in both physical and psychological health. Your adrenal glands are on your back, so you may have trouble reaching them. If so, first find the adrenals on the back of your partner or friend. To locate the adrenals, put your hand on your (or another person's) back and find the points of the shoulder blades on each side. Check the adrenal glands by placing your test magnet about 0.5 inch below the points of the shoulder blades.

5. Kidneys

The primary function of the kidneys is to regulate the composition and concentration of extracellular fluids, which surround every cell in your body. They form urine and deliver it to the urinary bladder where it is excreted. Many waste products are thus eliminated from the body. There are also useful products in the urine that the kidneys reabsorb.

Another very important duty of the kidneys is to keep blood from becoming too acidic. In our modern society, excess acid in our organs and tissues is almost universal. It is a major contributor to disease. When blood becomes very acidic (pH below 7.0), death occurs.

A major mission of the kidneys is to remove this excess acid from our bodies. That's why urine is acid and why properly functioning kidneys are a major contributor to health.

Like the adrenals, the kidneys are also tested on your back, on the right and left nipple line, around the belt line area for most people. Anatomically, this would be at the level of the bottom of the bottom (twelfth) rib. Because the adrenal glands sit on top of the kidneys, be sure to check low for the kidneys and high for the adrenals.

6. Thyroid Gland

The thyroid gland consists of two lobes. We test both lobes with our test magnet. Thyroid hormones create your metabolism rate, the speed with which your body transforms nutrients into energy. They also regulate our rate of growth and aging. A properly functioning thyroid gland is a major producer of health. An improperly functioning thyroid is a major producer of disease.

Another thyroid hormone increases the amount of calcium in the blood. It works with the parathyroid gland hormone, which decreases the amount of calcium in the blood, to insure that blood calcium is in balance.

To find the thyroid gland feel, on either side of your neck, for the thick, rope-like sternocleidomastoid muscle described earlier. In the middle of the rope, at the level of the bottom of your adam's apple, is where you check the thyroid gland. Check both the right and left sides separately.

7. Parathyroid Glands

These are four tiny glands, about the size of an apple seed, located on the posterior surface of the thyroid gland. As mentioned previously, the parathyroid glands provide a hormone that decreases the amount of calcium in the blood. Correct blood calcium requires both the thyroid and parathyroid glands to be working correctly and in balance.

The parathyroid glands also help bring about the reabsorption of calcium from the kidneys and intestines. They do this by activating vitamin D in the body.

The parathyroid glands can be found by placing your fingers on your clavicle or collar bone where it begins at the top of the sternum. Move your fingers sideways until you feel the beginning of the rope or SCM muscle. This will be about one inch on either side of your sternum or breastbone. This is the area where you check the parathyroid. Come in low so as not to confuse the parathyroid glands with the thyroid, and check on both sides.

8. The Stomach

The walls of the stomach are very muscular. Their job is to break the food we eat down into tiny particles. The more we chew our food, the easier we make it for our stomach to do this.

The stomach also stores food until the small intestine is ready to receive it. The small intestine processes only a small amount of food at a time. The stomach prepares the food to be digested in the intestines and then stores it until the small intestine can take it.

To test the stomach follow your sternum (breastbone) down, as we did earlier in the chapter, until you feel the soft spot at the end of the breastbone. This is where you check for both the esophagus and stomach. The esophagus is the food tube that extends from the back of your tongue to your stomach. If you get only a north pole response here, the stomach is called *hypoactive*. If you get only a south pole response here, the stomach is *hyperactive*.

There may be times when, because the esophagus and stomach combine, you may be concerned that you've gotten an esophagus reading instead of a stomach reading from your test. If you have any doubt over whether you're checking only your stomach, move sideways to the left under the rib cage to the left nipple line. Test in this area. If you get the same reading as you got before, it verifies the original stomach reading.

9. Hiatal Hernia

When you chew or swallow food it goes from your mouth into your esophagus, a tube that leads to your stomach. To get to your stomach the esophagus goes through an opening or hole in the diaphragm, the dome shaped muscle that separates your chest (where your ribs are) from your abdomen (which contains your stomach and intestines). The hole in the diaphragm is called the *esophageal hiatus.*

This is the point where the trouble begins. The stomach should be at all times below the diaphragm but in a Hiatal hernia, a part of the stomach goes up through the esophageal hiatus. This strongly contributes to acid reflux, or heartburn. Acid from the stomach now gets into the esophagus where the epithelium (skin layer of the esophagus) is damaged by the acid. This can create a condition called *Barrett's epithelium,* which can lead to cancer. Hiatal hernias are important because they can cause acid reflux and ultimately lead to esophageal cancer.

The test for the Hiatal hernia is the same as the stomach test above. If you get a response that is both north and south in the midline stomach area you have a Hiatal hernia.

10. Thymus Gland

The thymus gland produces cells called T-lymphocytes. Lymphocytes are white blood cells and are an important part of the immune system. A healthy, functioning thymus is required for healthy function of the immune system.

The thymus gland is large in a newborn child but decreases as we get older. Stimulation of the thymus can be a great help in treating bacterial infections and cancer.

Put your finger in the depression in your throat at the top of the breastbone. Check for the thymus on the midline, about 2 ribs or 1 inch down from the top of the breastbone.

11. Spleen

The spleen is part of the lymphatic and immune systems. The immune system operates through cells of the lymphatic system. The cells and products of the immune system are carried through lymphatic vessels and organs like the spleen.

The spleen is a storage depot for B-lymphocytes (lymphocytes from bone) and T-lymphocytes (lymphocytes from the thymus gland) that are the key cells of our immune system. It also filters the blood. When red blood cells break down they send iron to the liver where it is recycled.

The spleen is tested directly down from your arm pit on the left side of your body, about three ribs up from the lowest rib.

12. Uterus

The uterus is also called the womb. It contains and nourishes the human fetus from conception to birth. To test the uterus, locate the top of the pubic symphysis and move up so you're halfway between the pubic symphysis and the navel. This is the area to test the uterus.

13. Ovaries

There are two ovaries in the human female. They secrete two hormones, estrogen and progesterone that are responsible for female development. They also produce ova, or eggs, that develop into new human beings in the uterus when fertilized by male sperm.

To find the ovarian test area, find the pubic symphysis again. This is at the top of your hip bone where the two sides join. Do not go up from this area. Move your hand laterally (sideways) to the right and left nipple lines. These are the areas in which to test the left and right ovaries.

14. Prostate Gland

The prostate gland manufactures the fluid in which sperm cells float. The fluid made by the prostate is slightly alkaline, which neutralizes the acidity of the vagina, so the sperm can be mobile.

The prostate gland also stimulates the production of the hormone testosterone in the testes. Testosterone helps rebuild flabby muscles, stimulate brain cells, nourish the heart muscle and bring about renewed muscle tone throughout the body.

The prostate gland lies roughly between the rectum and the testes. Check for the prostate gland by moving down from the top of the pubic symphysis, halfway toward the penis. If you have any doubts over whether you might be checking the urinary bladder instead, confirm the reading by checking between the legs just above the rectum. If you get a similar reading to the one you got at the first site, you have confirmed the original reading.

15. Urinary Bladder

The kidney delivers urine to the urinary bladder, which then excretes it. The test site for the urinary bladder is on the midline (the pubic symphysis) just above the penis.

16. Colon

The importance of the colon may be judged from the fact that all your organs are connected to it and that their function is affected by the condition of your colon. The colon reabsorbs water, as well as vitamins, nutrients and toxic materials. Most notably, it compacts the materials not digested by the body into solid fecal matter.

In the colon, bacterial fermentation decomposes carbohydrates. Protein decomposition takes place by putrefaction. These processes produce very toxic products. If these toxins remain in the colon they are absorbed. Keeping feces in the colon excessively long can produce as many as 36 poisons.

One of the greatest health risks a person can take is to allow remnants of fermenting and putrefying food to remain in contact with the lining of the colon for three or more days. Failure to defecate also weakens the musculature of your colon. Your colon must have daily exercise and detoxification to remain strong and healthy. Constipation constitutes a major health problem and if it is present, any health program should *begin* with its correction.

The colon consists of an "ascending colon," which runs up the right side of the body, a "transverse colon" which crosses over to the left side, and a "descending colon" which goes down to the rectum on the left side of your body. The ascending colon is checked at a point slightly higher than the descending colon.

To find these points, move your hand down from your bottom ribs until you find the top of your hip bones. Keep feeling that bone and move down about 1 inch below the top of your hip bone on the right side and 2 to 3 inches below the top of your hip bone on the left. Now, on each side, move in to just about the nipple lines. This is where you will check your ascending colon on the right side and descending colon on the left. In most people today the transverse colon is prolapsed (has fallen down) so we can't find it and don't check it.

17. Diverticulitis

When the colon muscles get weak, sac-like outpocketings of the colon occurs. Undigested food collects in these outpocketings leading to irritation and inflammation. If in checking the colon you get a response to both the north and south pole, you have diverticulitis. Inflammation is registered by the south pole. Irritation is registered by the north.

Like constipation, diverticulitis should be immediately corrected.

18. Pituitary Gland

The pituitary is a pea-sized structure weighing about one-fifth of an ounce in an adult. It is suspended from the brain by a slender stalk located just above the back of the nose. It has two lobes: anterior and posterior.

The anterior lobe produces human growth hormone (HGH), one of the major growth-stimulating hormones in the body. The anterior lobe also produces hormones that stimulate the thyroid gland and adrenal cortex (adrenal glands). Other hormones stimulate milk production and ovulation in the female and testosterone production in the male.

The posterior lobe of the pituitary gland stores two important hormones originating in the hypothalamus. The hypothalamus is a major area of the brain that controls the activity of our autonomic nervous system—the part of our nervous system that regulates activities not under conscious control. The hormones are vasopressin and oxytocin.

The pituitary is checked on the midline, between the eyes, above the bridge of the nose where the eyebrows come together.

19. Pineal Gland

The pineal is a small gland that secretes a hormone called melatonin. Melatonin is believed to regulate the secretion of many other hormones and influence sleep-waking cycles.

The pineal gland is checked at the soft spot in the middle of the top of the head.

20. Heart

The heart is one of the toughest muscles in the human body and one of the most powerful and amazing pump systems in the world. It is about the size of a clenched fist and propels blood through an estimated 60,000 miles of blood vessels, pumping 3,500 gallons per day.

The left side of the heart pumps blood into the arteries. Arterial blood carries oxygen and nutrients. From the arteries, oxygen and nutrients go into the interstitial fluids (the fluids around body cells) and the cells of your body. In the veins, which carry blood back to the heart, tissue waste and carbon dioxide is added to the blood. The blood from the veins goes through the lungs, gives off its carbon dioxide and wastes, and takes on oxygen. This oxygen is then returned to the heart where it is sent out again by the arteries. In this way, the heart continually works to reoxygenate blood and send it through the body.

The proper function of the heart is critical to health and survival. The heart controls most of the electricity in the body. To find the test sites for the heart, locate the sternum. At the top, feel the first rib. Move down to between the second and third ribs. Testing is done in this area on both to the left of the sternum and to the right of the sternum. This measures the right and left auricles (upper chambers) of the heart. Next, move downward to the space between the fourth and fifth ribs. There, on both sides of the sternum, you test the ventricles (lower chambers) of the heart.

21. Lungs

The lungs are a pair of organs occupying most of the space in your chest. The lungs have the densest congregation of capillaries in the body so they can load oxygen into the blood. The trillions of cells in our body require a huge amount of oxygen, which is supplied by the lungs.

Testing the lungs is relatively simple. Everything in the chest that is not heart is lungs. The chest is above the diaphragm (the muscles and tendons that separate the chest and abdominal cavity). The lungs can be tested in the middle of the right and left side of the chest, away from the heart.

22. Blood

Circulating through every organ and tissue in your body, blood participates in every major element of body function. It is the stream of life.

Blood serves as a transport system for the body. It is the way nourishment, oxygen, hormones and other life essentials are carried to tissues of the body. It also transports waste products resulting from metabolic processes to the kidneys, skin, intestines and liver. Blood also clots as needed. Blood chemistry can tell us a great deal about how the body is functioning.

The blood is checked at the carotid artery bifurcation (branching) on the right side of the neck. Feel for the sternocleidomastoid muscle on the right side of your neck as you did when searching for the thyroid gland. Follow it upward with your fingers until you feel the bottom of your lower jaw. Under your jaw and in front of the SCM muscle, feel with your fingers until you feel the pulse of the carotid artery. The highest point at which you feel the carotid artery pulse is where to check the blood.

This is where the carotid artery bifurcates (branches). You check the carotid bifurcation on the right side of the neck to determine if the blood is normal, acid or alkaline.

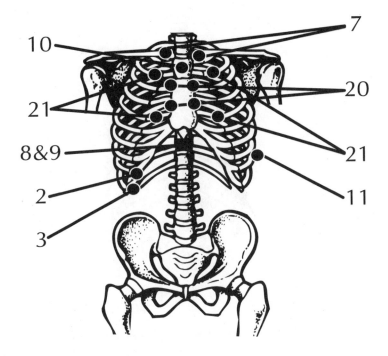

Test Points - Anterior View - Skeleton

2 Liver	8 Stomach	11 Spleen
3 Gall bladder	9 Hiatal hernia	20 Heart
7 Parathyroid gland	10 Thymus gland	21 Lungs

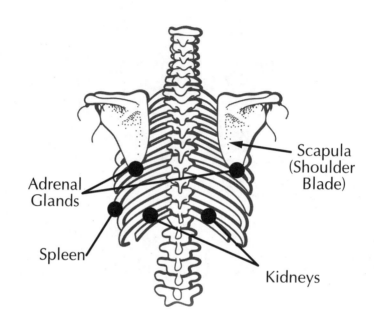

Adrenal Glands

Spleen

Scapula
(Shoulder
Blade)

Kidneys

Test Points - Posterior View - Skeleton

4 Adrenal glands   5 Kidneys   11 Spleen

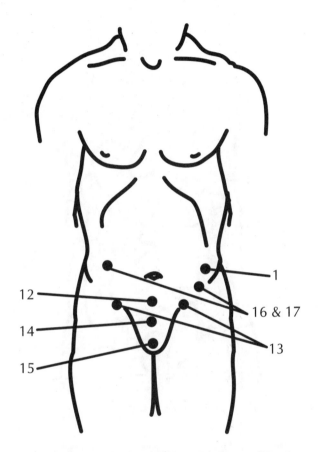

Test Points - Anterior View - Surface of Body

1 Pancreas	14 Prostate gland	16 & 17 Diverticulitis
12 Uterus	15 Urinary bladder	
13 Ovaries	16 & 17 Colon	

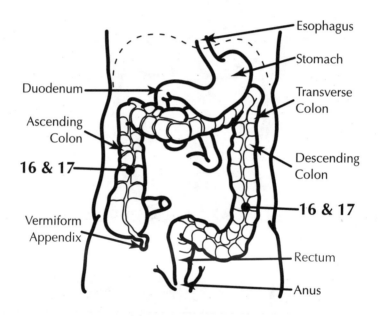

Esophagus

Stomach

Transverse
Colon

Duodenum

Ascending
Colon

Descending
Colon

16 & 17

16 & 17

Vermiform
Appendix

Rectum

Anus

Test Points - Colon

16 & 17 Colon   16 & 17 Diverticulitis

Two or even three readings can be made on the colon.

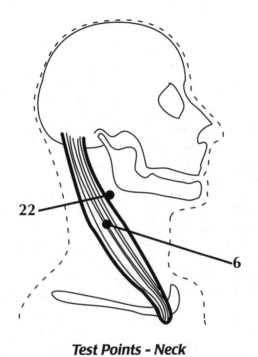

Test Points - Neck

6 Thyroid gland   22 Blood

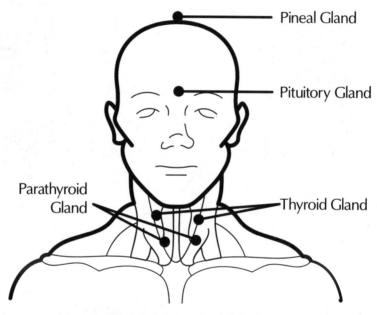

Pineal Gland

Pituitory Gland

Parathyroid Gland

Thyroid Gland

Test Points - Head and Neck

6 Thyroid gland	18 Pituitary gland
7 Paraathyroid gland	19 Pineal gland

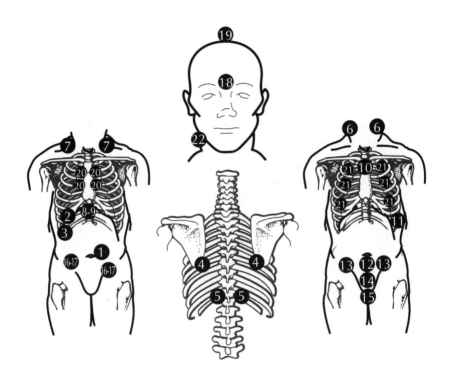

REACTION	REACTION	REACTION
__1. Pancreas	__8. Stomach	__15. Urinary Bladder
__2. Liver	__9. Hiatal Hernia	__16. Colon
__3. Gall Bladder	__10. Thymus Gland	__17. Diverticulitis
__4. Adrenal Glands	__11. Spleen	__18. Pituitary Gland
__5. Kidneys	__12. Uterus	__19. Pineal Gland
__6. Thyroid Gland	__13. Ovaries	__20. Heart
__7. Parathyroid Gland	__14. Prostrate Gland	__21. Lungs
		__22. Blood

South Pole is HYPER Active
North Pole is HYPO Active

CHAPTER 12

The Fundamentals–How to Correct Imbalances and Maintain Biohealth

A boy and a girl making love under a tanned haycock are far better employed than any military leader, be he ever so victorious.

—Llewelyn Powys, *Impassioned Clay*

Do you have the desire and strength of character to take responsibility for your own health?

Most people don't. They'd rather leave it all up to a doctor. Many people today still don't follow a healthy diet or exercise plan. They have totally separated themselves from their body yet they expect their body to take care of itself. If something goes wrong, hey, there's always the doctor. For these people, health begins after illness sets in.

Modern medicine plays right into this mentality. The emphasis today is on treating disease. Little or nothing is done to correct the cause of that disease. That is why we have so many chronic diseases that occur or recur after so-called "successful" treatment.

157

This is not to say that diseases shouldn't be treated or medical technology used. Medicine does great things. There are diseases that require medical treatment. But you should not use the treatment of a disease as a means for ignoring or failing to remove the root causes of a disease.

The Biohealth System strives to achieve four goals:

1. To correct the problem
2. To remove the root causes of any health problem by balancing the bioenergy fields and creating an environment within the body which, like a healthy soil, will grow only health
3. To enable the body to maintain its own health
4. To empower people to take responsibility for their own health

The Biohealth System takes commitment and even courage on your part. You don't just sit back and let somebody else take responsibility for your health and assume the scapegoat role when things don't go well. With Biohealth you no longer are a passive spectator of your own life and health. Biohealth requires that you take control. If you've got the desire and character to take responsibility for your own health, and only if you've got that desire and character, the Biohealth System is for you.

This chapter gives you the nuts and bolts of the Biohealth System. Magnetic testing tells you where you have a disease-producing field and where you have a health-producing field. The aim of the Biohealth System is not to destroy the disease and leave the disease-producing field intact. It is to replace the disease-producing bioenergy fields with health-producing bioenergy fields.

What Biohealth Students Experience

My former colleague Dr. Richard Broeringmeyer was a disciple of Albert Roy Davis, whose work we discussed in Chapter 6. Dr. Broeringmeyer often said he didn't have patients but students. And these were not even students of his: *They were students of their own body and of the energy that created them.*

He did not see his "students" on an individual basis but gave workshops in which groups were trained in the principles of Biohealth. Dr. Broeringmeyer understood that you are your own best teacher and your body is your best textbook.

And that's the bottom line in Biohealth. It can't be obtained solely by medical procedures. You are not a patient. You are a student of yourself and the energy that created you. You run the show. Biohealth involves returning your entire body to its highest functioning level. This happens when you get your bioenergy, the energy of your essence, in balance.

Understanding The Correcting Magnet, Also Called the Energy-Balancing Magnet

We learned earlier when using the test magnet that if the arm goes weak on one pole it goes strong on the other pole. When the arm goes weak, there is an energy field imbalance within the organ being tested and the test magnet makes that imbalance worse. The other pole makes the arm strong because it begins to correct the imbalance. This is the key to the correcting magnet. It provides a bigger, stronger version of what the test magnet does with the opposite pole.

The correcting magnet is the focus of the second step of the Biohealth System. Step 2 begins the process of restoring bioenergy balance. The reason that an organ is not balanced is that your body has lost its ability to balance it itself. The correcting magnet steps in to lend a hand where the body can't by supplying a charge opposite to what is in excess in the bioenergy field. When applied, it begins to balance or "correct" the existing unbalanced bioenergy field.

There are two types of energy-balancing magnets. The first is a flat rectangular magnet 4 inches long by 2 inches wide by 0.5 inch thick. It has a strength of 3,700 to 4,000 gauss, much

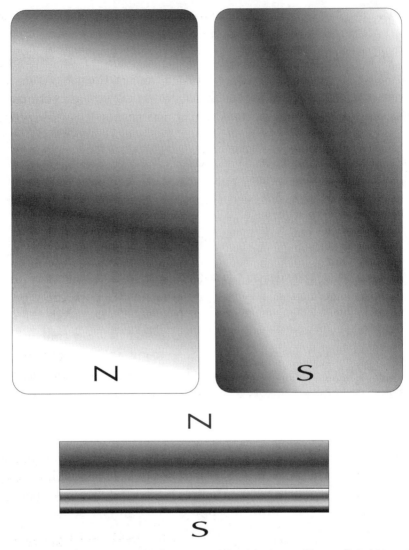

Energy Balancing Magnet: Flat magnets, 2 by 4 inches, with one flat side north pole and the other side south pole.

more than the testing magnet. One flat 2 by 4 inch side of the energy balancing magnet is a north pole and the other is a south pole. This allows you to place either the north or south pole over the organ being balanced as needed.

To balance an organ you use the pole that made the arm strong, the pole opposite to the one that made the arm weak.

160

The pole that made the arm strong is called the correcting or the balancing pole.

The balancing pole is placed directly over the organ being balanced. As long as the balancing pole is over the organ, the bioenergy is being balanced. A second balancing magnet is placed over the top of the first one. The main reason for the second balancing magnet is to hold the first one in place. The second magnet also increases the gauss, but since it is more than 0.5 inch away from the body, it will deliver less than its 3,700 gauss to the organ being balanced. But there is still a cumulative effect on the organ being corrected.

Here's how it works: Suppose you are balancing your pancreas, and you have a south pole pancreas. You know that the pancreas is located where your left nipple line crosses your belly button line, so you place the north pole of the correcting magnet over that area to balance the south pole imbalance. As mentioned earlier, since wearing the magnet a long time might irritate the skin, you can prevent this by placing a thin garment— such as a T-shirt or undershirt—between the magnet and the skin.

The second magnet will hold the correcting magnet in place. The second correcting magnet is called a "holding" magnet, because its primary purpose is to hold the correcting magnet in place over the organ being balanced. You place the holding magnet over the correcting magnet with both north poles facing the pancreas.

Since the correcting magnet has its north pole facing the pancreas, its south pole is facing away from the pancreas. You now put on a garment that covers the correcting magnet. When the holding magnet is placed with its north pole also facing the pancreas, the north pole of the holding magnet comes into contact with the south pole of the correcting magnet. They strongly attract each other. This attraction between the south pole of the correcting magnet and the north pole of the holding magnet, with a garment between them, will firmly hold the magnets in place.

You're left with a configuration like this: T-shirt, correcting magnet (north pole down), garment and holding magnet (north pole down). The magnetic attraction of the opposite poles with the garment between them will hold the magnets in place.

. You can also wear the correcting magnets on a jacket, as shown in the photo, or over any clothing. Since the main correcting magnetic energy is from the balancing magnet, the fact that the holding magnet is slightly farther from the organ being balanced will have little significance.

HOLDING THE ENERGY BALANCING MAGNET IN PLACE.

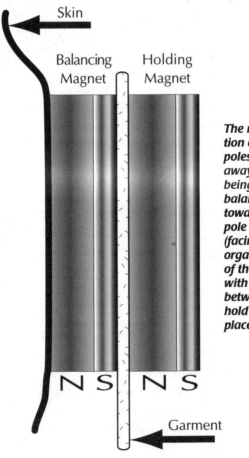

The magnetic attraction of the opposite poles of the top (facing away from the organ being corrected) of the balancing magnet toward the opposite pole of the bottom (facing toward the organ being corrected) of the holding magnet with a garment between them will hold the magnets in place.

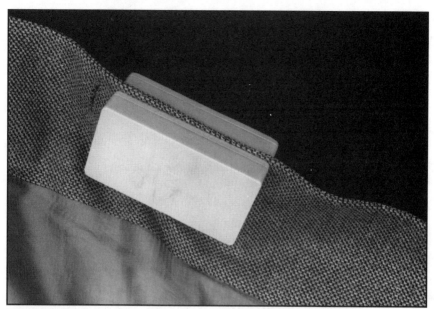

Balancing magnet and holding magnet with garment between them.

The Super Magnet

The second type of magnet is both a correcting and stimulating magnet. It is a smaller but a much more powerful magnet. It has the amazing power of 12,500 gauss. For that reason it is called a "super magnet."

The super magnet has a diameter of only 1 inch and is 0.4 inch thick but packs super magnetic energy. With the super magnet you purchase another small round magnet of 1 inch diameter and 3,800 gauss, which matches the size of the super magnet. It is the holding magnet of the super magnet. It fits above it and holds the super magnet in place exactly the same as the 2 by 4 magnets described previously.

Super magnets are also made with a pouch. This pouch has strings attached to it that can tie the magnet in place over almost any area of the body. The super magnet can be used without the round magnet in this case, increasing the convenience of the super magnet.

163

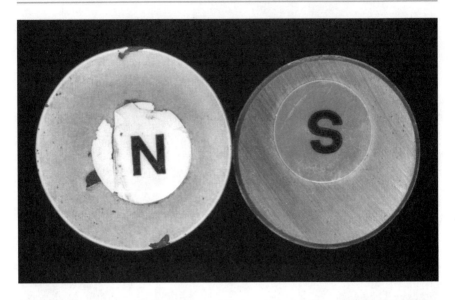

The super magnet is new. The rectangular correcting magnets have been used for many years. Because of their much greater convenience, the super magnets are now being used more for balancing than the 2 by 4 correcting magnet. There is an enormous amount of documentation as to the effectiveness of the 2 by 4 balancing magnet. At this time, there is not as much data on the super magnet.

In cancer and with infections it is very important to stimulate the immune system. In fact, in today's society it is almost universally important to stimulate the immune system. By doing this you stimulate the thymus gland. That is done only with the super magnet. You place the super magnet with its south pole, its stimulating pole, over and facing the thymus gland and wear it for as many hours possible.

To stimulate the immune system you want a south pole reading on the thymus gland, and then keep the super magnet on it long enough to always get a thymus gland south pole reading.

The depth a magnet will penetrate into the body depends more on size than gauss strength, The 2 by 4 inch rectangular magnet covers a larger area and penetrates deeper than the super magnet. If you are using a super magnet for correcting and you're not getting the desired results, you may need more penetration, so switch to the 2 by 4 magnets.

When dealing with problems like cancer and infections, where deep penetration and large coverage are needed, use only the 2 by 4 magnets. (Cancer will be covered in more detail in Chapter 14.)

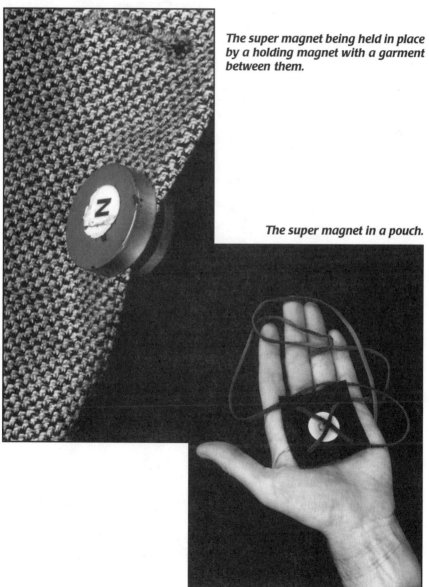

The super magnet being held in place by a holding magnet with a garment between them.

The super magnet in a pouch.

SUPER MAGNET - Actual Size

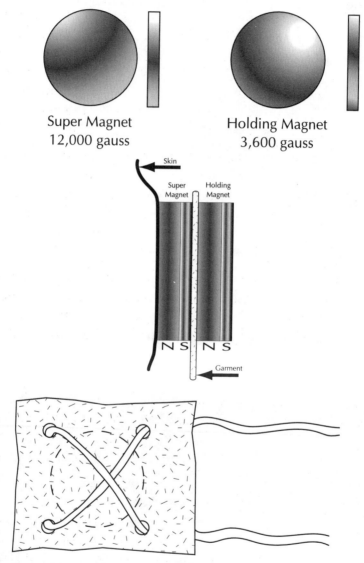

Super Magnet
12,000 gauss

Holding Magnet
3,600 gauss

Super Magnet in a pouch with strings to tie it in place.

The super magnet can be used with a holding magnet to attach it to a garment. It also comes in a pouch which can be tied anywhere.

Balancing Energy Fields Is Crucial to Achieving Health

It is important to know what you are accomplishing with the correcting magnets. When bioenergy fields are not balanced, organs do not function properly. Food, no matter how good, will not be fully metabolized. Unmetabolized food ferments and turns into acid. Waste products are not fully removed from the cell. Enzymes, which control chemical reactions in the cell, are not activated. The list of destructive effects goes on and on.

Thus, after testing, the first step in restoring correct function is to begin balancing the bioenergy fields. This will improve nutrition, enzyme function, hormone function, genetic function and the overall operation of your entire body. Without balanced bioenergy fields it is very difficult, and sometimes impossible, to achieve a health-producing environment.

The effect of the correcting magnet is quite remarkable. Once it is applied to any organ, gland or tissue that has a bioenergy imbalance, its function immediately improves. As the bioenergy field of the organ is improved further, it begins to do its job again.

However—and this is important—it is still the correcting magnet that is balancing the field. It's not your body. When the magnet is removed, the bioenergy imbalance will still be there. The goal of the Biohealth System is to ultimately, at the end of the correction time, have your own body balance its magnetic fields.

When you remove the correcting magnet, you then test the organ with the testing magnet. As long as there is an imbalance, you keep using the correcting magnet. When you remove the correcting magnet and the testing magnet shows no imbalance, you have achieved biomagnetic, bioenergy balance, and health.

In step 7 of the Biohealth System we prove whether your body can restore a bioenergy imbalance. This is very important

167

because if you have not corrected the cause of the problem, it and other problems can recur.

Now, step-by-step, here is the complete Biohealth System.

Step 1–Testing

You already know how to do this, and hopefully you have purchased your magnets and are doing it.

Step 2–Restoring Bioenergy Balance

If you get a positive south pole test reading on an organ, you correct with the north pole of the correcting magnet. If you get a positive north pole test reading on an organ, you correct with the south pole of the correcting magnet. The correcting magnets should be used for a minimum of three hours, but they must not be overused. They are used until the organ being corrected is in balance. It is in balance when you remove the correcting magnet and there is no reading on either the north or south pole of the test magnet.

What happens if you use the correcting magnet too long? How do you know what is too long? When you use the magnet too long you create an imbalance toward the correcting pole of the magnet. If you are using the south pole to balance an organ, and you get a south pole reading, switch to the north pole. Check it every day, and in a short time it will be back in balance. Checking makes it impossible to create a magnetic imbalance.

In order to become an expert with the testing magnet, we suggest you check all 22 test points described in Chapter 10.

Once you can test reliably, the next step is to correct. As described previously, this involves placing the proper pole of the correcting magnet over the organ you are balancing.

How do you choose which unbalanced organs to balance first? It's best to begin correcting with the five major organs:

1. Kidneys

2. Pancreas

3. Liver

4. Adrenal glands

5. Heart

We've found that when you balance the five major organs, most of the other unbalanced organs in the body will become balanced. We've also found that if we balance other organs, and we do not have the five majors balanced, the balance in the other organs won't hold. The five majors lead the way. Therefore, the first step is to balance the five major organs.

Begin by placing the correct balancing magnetic field over each of the majors that is unbalanced. If necessary, balance all five. If more than one or two requires balancing, we've usually found it best to use the super magnet because they can easily be worn and the 2 by 4 magnets are heavy and bulky.

An additional important note. If, along with any of the above five, you get an imbalance reading on the colon, you should detoxify and clean out the colon along with the five. With a colon out of balance, it can be difficult to balance the five majors. So, with an imbalance reading in the colon, add it to the five. *Important: If the colon is out of balance or has diverticulitis, treat the colon along with the 5 majors.*

When Not to Do the Five Major First

There are two situations when the five majors are not done first. One of these occasions involves infection. With an infection, before anything else, you want to stop the bacteria from proliferating. What pole slows down life? The north pole. With an infection you place the north pole of the correcting magnet over the infected area. This weakens and stops the growth of bacteria. Always treat an infection before you do the five majors.

Note: Never put a south pole over an infected area. The south pole is the magnetic energy of life. It enhances and increases all life but does not distinguish between good and bad. Put a south pole over an infected area and you will increase the number of toxic bacteria and the toxic strength of the bacteria.

Along with weakening and stopping the growth of bacteria, there is another thing you want to do with an infection: Raise the immune system to its highest level. With an infection, you can be sure your immune system needs strengthening. After all, if it was at its highest level you probably wouldn't even have the infection!

In the Biohealth System, we strengthen the immune system by stimulating the thymus gland and balancing the thymus. We stimulate the thymus gland by placing the south pole of the super magnet over it. As mentioned above, the super magnet is especially effective in stimulating the thymus gland and I prescribe using it routinely. The super magnet usually will balance the spleen. If it does not, switch to the correcting magnet.

With infections it's always north pole over the infected area, south pole over the thymus gland, and balance the spleen.

The second situation that requires immediate attention is cancer. All cancers are strongly south pole. With cancer, the first requirement is to stop the growth of the cancer. The north pole does this. When treating cancer, placing a north pole on the cancer along with a south pole over the thymus, and balancing the spleen is an immediate priority.

Note: Never place a south pole over a cancer. It will make it more powerful. It will grow faster.

Length of Treatment

As we've pointed out many times already, people are unique. Each is different from every other. There is probably no more important principle in any health system.

Diseases are also different. Some are more severe than others. As a result, there is no standard duration of time for wearing the correcting magnet each day. The main thing you need to do is to keep checking the organ. If the organ becomes neutral, neither north nor south pole, you know you've done the job.

There are some general rules, however. Obviously, if you're dealing with something life threatening like a cancer, you'll want to wear the correcting magnet 12 hours or more a day. If you're dealing with something of lesser severity, you may wear the magnet less.

In the end, it all comes down to *testing, testing, testing*. If you see you're not getting what you want, you wear the correcting magnet more. Listen to your body and continue to use the correcting magnet until it says you are in control.

By testing, you put yourself in the position of always knowing what your condition is and what you need to do. When an organ reaches balance, you stop. If the organ moves beyond its balanced position, you'll know you've overdone it, and you easily correct it.

The main thing with the correcting magnet is not how long you wear it. It's checking to see if you're getting the results you want. You can check the organ at the end of every day, every week or every month. When it's where you want it to be, you have achieved bioenergy balance. It's that simple. The important thing is to keep checking.

Step 3—Stopping the Autoimmune Attack

Now that we've tested (step 1) and begun to restore bioenergy balance (step 2) we're ready to move on to step 3 in the Biohealth System. In step 3 we stop the autoimmune attack on the malfunctioning organ.

In 1947, Dr. Royal Lee published a revolutionary book titled *Protomorphology*. This book asserted that when organs malfunction and/or become diseased, the body regards them as foreign objects and produces antibodies that attack them. Put simply, this means the body attacks its own organs. This an *autoimmune attack*. The antibodies your body produces attack its own organs. Dr. Lee called these antibodies *natural tissue antibodies*.

At the time the book was published it was violently denounced by the medical profession but subsequent research has proven Lee correct. An autoimmune attack has been shown to be a part of virtually all disease processes.

This is important to the Biohealth System. For all practical purposes, you can assume that an organ whose energy is out of balance will simultaneously experience an autoimmune attack. Along with balancing the organ's bioenergy, stopping this autoimmune attack is very important to restoring health.

While studying the autoimmune response, Dr. Lee discovered something very interesting and important. When an organ was under attack, he took a piece of that same organ from an animal and put it in tablet form so it could be taken orally and end up in the blood stream. When the remains of the animal organ appeared in the blood stream, the natural tissue antibodies attacked it and left the diseased organ alone. He called the tablet containing the animal organ a protomorphogen (PMG).

PMGs have subsequently proven an invaluable part of our program for balancing bioenergy. As an example, suppose you were testing your spleen and found it to be malfunctioning with either a north or south pole reading. In this situation, you can almost be sure the spleen is under an autoimmune attack so you take a piece of the spleen from an animal in the form of a PMG. Your natural tissue antibodies would then attack the PMG in the bloodstream and stop attacking your spleen allowing it time to heal and return to balance and proper function.

PMGs are produced by a company called Standard Process. 23 PMGs are now available. Following is a list of these PMGs and the organs with which they are associated:

PMG	Organ
Biost PMG	Bone marrow, spinal cord
Cardiotrophin PMG	Heart
Dermatrophin PMG	Epithelial tissue, skin
Drenatrophin PMG	Adrenal glands
Hepatrophin PMG	Liver
Hypothalamus PMG	Hypothalamus
Mammary PMG	Mammary glands, breasts
Myotrophin PMG	Heart muscle
Neurotrophin PMG	Brain
Oculotrophin PMG	Eye
Orchic PMG	Testis
Ostrophin PMG	Bone marrow, spinal cord
Ovatrophin PMG	Ovaries
Pancreatrophin PMG	Pancreas
Parotid PMG	Parotid gland
Pituitrophin PMG	Pituitary gland
Pneumotrophin PMG	Lungs
Prostate PMG	Prostate
Renatrophin PMG	Kidneys
Spleen PMG	Spleen
Thymus PMG	Thymus
Thytrophin PMG	Thyroid gland
Utrophin PMG	Uterus

Whenever we place a balancing magnet over a malfunctioning organ (step 2) where it is available we simultaneously use the PMG of that organ (step 3). Steps 2 and 3 of the seven-step Biohealth System thus begin at the same time. They also end at the same time. *As long as use of the correcting magnet is indicated, you should continue taking the PMG to redirect any possible autoimmune attack.*

As you will see later in the chapter, once you restore biological health neither the magnet nor PMG are needed. In order to achieve biological health, however, both should be included in the process.

Organic Homeopathics

Homeopathic organ preparations can also stop autoimmune attacks. Because of this, if you're working with an organ or tissue that doesn't have a protomorphogen (PMG), a homeopathic organ remedy can also stop the autoimmune attack.

Unlike the PMG, which you simply take orally, homeopathic organotherapy is not something you can do. You need to find a homeopathic practitioner who has experience and training in organ therapy. Incorrectly used they can do harm, so you must seek the help of a homeopathic practitioner who knows homeopathic organotherapy.

Step 4—Determining the Correct Nutrition for You

There are five major factors that produce malfunction and disease that we focus on in the Biohealth System: (1) nutrition, (2) stress, (3) toxicity, (4) structural problems and (5) lack of exercise.

Disease, symptoms and malfunction are not really the problem. They are manifestations of the problem. The purpose of Biohealth is to determine the cause of the problem and correct that root cause so that the body can keep itself in health.

Each one of the factors above can be pivotal in creating an environment where disease can appear but nutrition is a key factor around which all the others revolve. Nutritional deficiencies can result from lack of nutrition, incorrect nutrition and the inability of the body to digest, assimilate and metabolize nutrients. Excluding genetic disease, we have found these nutritional deficiencies to be a basic factor in producing disease. Indeed, none of the other factors above can be corrected without proper nutrition.

This nutritional focus places us at step 4 in the Biohealth Program. We've tested (step 1), restored magnetic balance with the energy balancing magnet (step 2) and stopped the autoim-

174

mune attack with PMGs (step 3). Now we're ready to begin to supply our body with the nutrition it tells us it needs.

The Story of Remedy Testing

We need to ask a major question at this point. This question is absolutely essential to Biohealth: How do you know, not guess, what nutrition your body needs?

The late nutritionist Dr. Roger J. Williams wrote a book titled *Biochemical Individuality* where he says that no two of us are alike and that the nutritional needs of no two people are identical. What helps another person with the "same" problem may not help you. What statistically, in double-blind studies, helps most people may actually harm you. Each of us needs an individual nutritional program designed for our needs alone.

How do we create such a program? How do we determine the nutritional needs of our bodies without guesswork and doubt? We ask our body what it needs. Thanks to the clinical genius of Dr. Reinhold Voll of Germany, and a little serendipity (which always seems to play a role in science and research), we know how to do this.

Dr. Voll was an expert in electroacupuncture and developed an instrument called the *dermatron*. He treated patients using the dermatron and homeopathic remedies. He also gave workshops for physicians only.

At one workshop, just before lunch, he tested a physician and found that his prostate gland was malfunctioning. He told the group that, after lunch, he'd show them how to correct the prostate gland. After lunch Dr. Voll checked the physician's prostate again and to his surprise, it checked normal. Members of the audience, skeptics in good standing, immediately said that this showed that Dr. Voll's dermatron could be wrong but Dr. Voll stuck to his guns. He countered that he knew his machine was right and the physician must have done something over the lunch break to correct his prostate.

The audience laughed but Dr. Voll persisted and vowed to find out how the physician's prostate had been corrected. He questioned the doctor about what he'd done over lunch but found nothing that would affect his prostate gland.

Still Voll continued, his confidence unshaken. The workshop was taking place in the office of a homeopathic physician who had handed two homeopathic remedies used to treat the prostate gland to the doctor, who had in turn put them in his pocket. He told this to Dr. Voll and the class, and Dr. Voll asked him to take the two remedies out of his pocket.

When the doctor took those bottles out of his pocket, lo and behold, his prostate gland tested abnormal. But when he picked up the two bottles and placed them in his hand his prostate checked normal again.

Remedy testing had begun. The doctor's almost mindless pocketing of the bottles at lunch and Dr. Voll's persistence and self-belief had created an exciting, new tool for health.

Magnetic remedy testing is, today, one of the most powerful tools available for Biohealth. It tells you what any supplement or drug will do for your body before you take it. It allows you to take any substance and, before you even put it into your body, test it and know what it will do. It allows you to ask your body what it needs and get an answer.

There are two parts to remedy testing, both of which provide invaluable information. The first tells you if the remedy you're testing will help you or not. The second tells you the quantity or how much of the substance you should take for best results.

In the first part, we bring out the test magnet again. Before, we used it to determine if the energy in an organ was in balance or not. Now we use it as a means for our body to tell us what the correct nutrition is for us. When you bring a food or supplement into the energy field of the organ, the test magnet will tell you what effect that food or substance has on the organ's energy field.

For example, suppose we tested a person and found an alkaline (north pole) pancreas. Suppose we then put a food (or nutritional supplement, herb and so forth) into the electromagnetic field of the pancreas. When tested again, the pancreas tested balanced.

This tells us that whatever was put into the electromagnetic field of the pancreas will help restore the energy balance of the pancreas. Now we know that when the person ingests that substance, his or her body will use it to help restore functional health and bioenergy balance.

How do you put anything into the electromagnetic field of the body? It is simple. If a person holds the substance in his or her hand or puts it anywhere it touches the skin or is near the skin, the energy of the substance is transferred into the electromagnetic field of the body. It will then also be transferred into the pancreas or whatever organ you are testing.

To put anything into the electromagnetic field of an organ being tested, have the subject hold it in one of their hands or put it under their belt or anywhere where it is touching or near the skin. For food, place the food on a plate and have the subject hold the plate in their hand. Then you test the organ in question. If an unbalanced organ becomes balanced you have a healthy food, if a balanced organ becomes unbalanced you have an unhealthy food. There's no guesswork here.

That's one of the great things about magnetic testing. It is objective. We've found that the magnet gives us a totally objective reading that our beliefs cannot affect.

Magnetic testing is noninvasive. It has no side effects. It's totally harmless. Unlike medical and other tests that can be difficult and offer questionable application, magnetic testing is convenient, reliable and gives you immediate answers. It allows you to take control of your health, to take control of the functioning of your body and eventually take control of your life!

Remedy Testing–An Example

Let's take a look at a complete remedy testing example by adding the second and final part of the procedure—testing for quantity—to the equation. Suppose you are testing your pancreas and on the south pole your arm goes weak. You know at this point you have a south pole pancreas and you will need to use the correcting magnet and PMG. You also need to know what kind of nutrition will help restore balance to the pancreas so you begin to test supplements.

To test a supplement, hold the container of the substance in your hand. This puts it into the circuit of the pancreas. While you're still holding the substance, the pancreas is again tested with the south pole of the test magnet. If it is a supplement that will help correct the energy imbalance of the pancreas, the arm will become strong while you are holding that supplement.

Before, the arm went weak when the south pole of the test magnet was applied. Now, while holding the supplement and testing with the south pole, the arm is strong. The supplement is balancing the energy of the pancreas. You now know that when you take this supplement, it will be of benefit to you.

When you first start remedy testing, after the initial testing of a supplement, we urge you to put it down and test the pancreas again with the south pole. The arm will be weak. Then pick up the supplement again and test with the south pole. It will be strong. By repeating the test you'll add confidence and some real motivation if you're just beginning the Biohealth System. We now know (not guess or hope) this supplement will help restore energy balance to the pancreas. Your body, by its response to the food supplement, has told you this is so.

This can be a very empowering moment. To see the arm go weak on the test and find it strong when you do the same test with the supplement is very impressive. Almost without exception, when the subject sees this happen they are excited to go ahaead. We urge you to take a moment to really appreciate what you've done when you reach this point in the Biohealth process.

The second part of remedy testing involves answering questions about how much of the supplement or food a person should take. Again with the test magnet, you ask your body these questions and it will tell you. The test magnet has a direct private line to your inner body.

Here's how this works with the previous example. Assume your supplement comes in tablet form. Take one tablet out of the container, hold it in your hand and test the pancreas with the south pole, which had indicated an imbalance earlier. If the arm goes weak again, you know that's not enough of a dosage. You then take two tablets in your hand, test the pancreas with the south pole and find your arm is strong. Your body has told you that this is a correct dosage. Now take three tablets in your hand and test the pancreas with the south pole. If your arm goes weak, your body has told that is too much.

Through the use of the test magnet, your body tells you what you should give it and how much.

An important note: If your arm goes strong on two or more readings, say on both two and three tablets, you will use the larger amount to correct a more severe health problem. Use the smaller amount for supplementing smaller problems.

Food Testing

Tests can also be done on the food you eat. There are two ways to test foods under differing conditions. First, you have already been told how to know if a food will help to correct an imbalanced bioenergy field. You use the test magnet and the arm goes weak on, say, the south pole. You hold a plate of food and on the south pole, the arm does not go weak. You know this food will help correct the imbalance

There is a second test for foods that does not use magnetic testing. This test does not tell you if the food will help you, but it does tell you if the food will cause bioenergy imbalances in your body, which is important to know. This simple test can be done anywhere at any time. Simply, if you hold anything in or on your left hand, and someone presses on your right wrist and your right arm goes weak. Whatever you are holding in or on your left hand is producing bioenergy imbalances in your body.

This is often used to check foods in a grocery store. You hold a food in your left hand (in some people it may work better in the right hand, but in most the left hand is best) and have someone press on your right wrist. If the right arm goes down, that food is causing bioenergy imbalances in your body.

You can also check any foods you eat. Put them on a plate and hold the plate in your left hand, and if your right arm goes weak, that food is causing bioenergy imbalances. I do not recommend eating foods that cause bioenergy imbalances.

Time and again we have found a quantity of food that did not produce an energy imbalance, but when we added more of the same food to the plate the arm went weak. A larger quantity of the same food produced a bioenergy imbalance. Obviously, you do not eat that quantity of food. It is important to check for both quality and quantity.

It is possible for a plate or food container to cause a bioenergy imbalance. Therefore, before checking the food, check the plate or whatever you will put the food on. Hold the plate or container and see if the right arm goes weak. If it does, do not use that plate or container.

Liquids can be tested the same way. First check the container, then the liquid, and then the quantity of liquid. Limit your intake of liquids to those that do not cause bioenergy imbalances.

A word of caution: When you are not using a magnet always remember that what the person doing the testing believes, or any malfunction they have, can weaken the arm of the person being tested and produce a false result.

A Practical Food Testing Situation

I was fortunate to have studied nutrition with the late great Hazel Parcells for many years. One day I took her out to lunch. I was sure Hazel would choose a health food restaurant but she surprised me by choosing a fast food restaurant that specialized in fried fish.

She ordered fried fish and French fries. Being a good student, I made the same choice but I couldn't help questioning Hazel about it.

"What kind of nutrition is this?" I asked her.

"I like fried fish and french fries," she replied. "I've tested them and found that I can eat them once every four days and have no ill effects at all."

In fact, you don't have to be a total dietary bore to be healthy. By using testing, you can determine how often you can eat those unhealthy foods you enjoy with no ill effects. I've found I can eat a fudge chocolate sundae every fifth day with no ill effects.

Ain't testing wonderful!

Nutritional Needs Change

Your life is always in a state of change. With these changes, your nutritional needs may also change. With remedy testing, you can determine at any time what nutrition and supplements will balance your bioenergy and how much of them you will need. This is why learning how to test yourself is of critical importance. Nobody else but you and your body can do remedy testing.

Only you can monitor your health. That is the bottom line of the Biohealth System. In whatever situations arise in life, Biohealth gives you the ability to test the bioenergy balance of your organs and the nutritional needs of your body.

Health is not something you have or do not have. Health is something you do. Health is a dynamic, constantly changing process! That is why it is essential that you know how to test.

There are four other basic factors that may need correcting to get your body to a state of Biohealth. They are toxicity, stress, body structure and exercise. The important thing to remember is that without correct nutrition no magnet, no PMG, no stress control, no detoxification, no structural corrections and no exercise program will bring you to lasting health.

The Standard Process Supplements

Two little words form the answer to every health question you may have: Test it!

Biohealth remedy testing begins with a list of the 22 Biohealth test areas presented in the last chapter and the supplements associated with each test area. But this list is only a guide for your testing. Do not use the supplements listed because they have been successfully used by other people. The only way you can know which of these will help you is to test them. Use nothing until you test it.

You test them by performing the remedy testing procedure we've just discussed and finding out which of them will restore bioenergy balance to your unbalanced organs, glands and tissues.

The list below is for Standard Process supplements. Standard Process is a company in Wisconsin that uses whole food supplements that have no synthetics. Whole food supplements are much more potent than vitamins alone because they include enzymes and other important substances that vitamins alone do not have.

Nowhere in nature do vitamins occur in isolation. Nature has never learned how to produce vitamins in isolation. Only man has. Vitamins are parts of total food complexes. The only source of total food complexes is natural whole foods. All Standard Process supplements are whole food complexes.

You may use other companies as long as you test their supplements before using them. Since I use Standard Process the most and know them the best, they are what I will now share with you.

The following list below was created by Mark Anderson, an expert in using the standard process supplements, and it includes the Standard Process supplements I use the most. It is an excellent guide to what is available but, again, these must be tested before they're used. Whatever brand you use (and there are other fine brands), whatever supplements you use, they must all be tested before you use them. The goal is to create a nutrition that works for you.

Below you'll find each of our 22 Biohealth test areas with the Standard Process supplements associated with each. You can use the first two, or any two, of the listed supplements that you test. Two is usually all you will need. However, as long as you test it, you can use or any combination or amount.

Test Area	Supplements
1. Pancreas	Diaplex, Cataplex GTF, Cataplex B, Zypan, Multizyme, Zinc Liver Chelate
2. Liver	Livaplex, AF Betafood, Antronex, Chlorophyll, Complex Perles, Choline, Ferrofood, Chezyn, Allorganic Trace Minerals, Zinc Liver Chelate, Cataplex A, Cataplex B, Cataplex E, Magnesium Lactate, Organic Minerals
3. Gall bladder	AF Betafood, Cholacol, Choline, Livaplex
4. Adrenal glands	Drenamin, B_6 Niacinamide, Cataplex B, Cataplex C, Cataplex G, Proteofood, Organic Minerals
5. Kidneys and bladder	Arrginex, Renafood, Cataplex A, Phosfood Liquid, Cal-Ma Plus Cal-Amo, Calcium Lactate, Organic Minerals, Magnesium Lactate, Ferrofood

Test Area	Supplements
6. Thyroid gland	Organic Iodine, Iodomere, Cataplex C, Cataplex F, Antronex, Allorganic Trace Minerals, Min-Tran
7. Parathyroid gland lactate	Cal-Ma Plus, Cataplex D, Calcium
8. Stomach	Zypan, Betaine Hydrochloride,
9. Hiatal hernia	Gastrex, Okra Pepsin E3, Chlorophyll Complex Perles
10. Thymus gland	Thymex, Cataplex A-C, Cataplex ACP, Congaplex, Immuplex, Copper Liver Chelate
11. Spleen	Whole Disiccate Spleen, Chlorophyll Complex Perles, Immuplex, Chezyn, Ferrofood, Organic Minerals, Sesame Seed Oil
12. Uterus	The same as ovaries but with Utrophin PMG
13. Ovaries	Ovex, Wheat Germ Oil Perles, Chlorophyll Complex Perles, Organic Iodine, Iodomere, Cataplex E
14. Prostate gland	Prost-X, Zinc Liver Chelate, Cataplex F, Calcium Lactate, Organic Iodine
16. For both Colon and 17. Diverticulitis	Lact-Enz, Zymex, Zymex II, Lactic Acid Yeast, Okra-Pepsin E3, Gastrex, Cataplex C, Livaplex, Spanish Black Radish
18. Pituitary gland	Cataplex E, Manganese-B$_{12}$, E-Manganese
19. Pineal gland	Folic Acid B$_{12}$, Neuroplex, Cataplex C, Sunlight and Natural UV Radiation

Test Area	Supplements
20. Heart	Cardio-Plus, Myo-Plus, Cataplex E, Vasculin, Calcium Lactate, Cal-Ma Plus, Cataplex B, Cataplex C, Cataplex E, Cataplex F, Cataplex G, Organic Minerals, Phosfood Liquid, Linum B_6
21. Lungs	Cataplex A-C, Cataplex ACP, Emphaplex, Calcium Lactate, Cal-Ma Plus, Calsol, Cataplex F, Allerplex, Cogngaplex, Antronex, Fen-Gre, Phosfood, Drenamin, Manganese-B_{12}
22. Blood	Chlorophyll Complex Perles, Cataplex B_{12}, Folic Acid B_{12}, For-Til B_{12}, Calcium Lactate, Cal-Ma Plus, Calsol, Sesame Seed Oil, Ferrofood, Linum B_6, Chezyn, Organic Materials, Copper Liver Chelate, Zinc Liver Chelate, Phosfood Liquid, Soy Bean Lecithin

There are many supplements here but Standard Process fortunately has a test kit that allows us to test these supplements and choose the correct ones without breaking our wallets. The test kit consists of 135 substances.

You will also notice that the same supplement can be used for different areas. If you find a supplement that applies to more than one area, that is fine. Use it for both areas. Usually you will not have to use more than two supplements for an area. When you use more than one supplement, be sure to check them both individually and together with all other supplements being used. It does not matter how many or how few supplements you use as long as you test them. The Standard Process supplement can only be purchased from health professionals. Call Standard Process for names.

On average, it takes about three to four months for supplements to work, so be patient. Whatever the situation, your testing

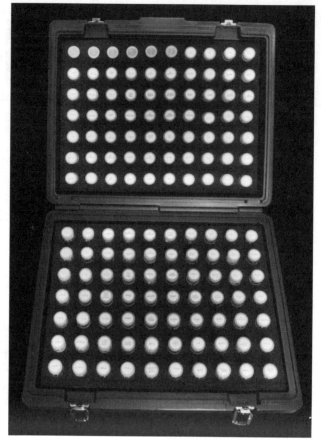

The standard process test kit.

magnet will ultimately tell you when you've achieved balance and you're ready to suspend the supplement or readjust how much of the supplement you're taking.

Protomorphogens and Testing

PMGs are not included on the list above but for every organ that has a PMG, you should take the PMG.

You cannot magnetically test PMGs. PMGs are like money to a starving man. You give a starving man a steak to hold in his hand and he tests it. The test will show that he needs the steak. But when you give him a $100 bill and he tests it, the test shows he doesn't need it. A paper $100 bill will not restore bioenergy balance. But you can buy a lot of steak with that $100.

PMGs are like the $100 bill. They aren't the steak but they allow you to buy the steak. Since the PMG itself doesn't correct the energy imbalance it often won't test as being needed. But, since it stops the concurrent autoimmune attack, it is important. Whether they test needed or not, every organ out of balance needs its PMG. Energy balance is more difficult to restore without PMGs.

The amount of PMG you should take is, again, up to you. Too many will not harm, but they do no more good than the correct amount.

Step 5—Applying and Monitoring the Biohealth Program

We've now provided you with a program for restoring balanced bioenergy to any organ, gland or tissue. We have discussed the need for testing (step 1), restoring bioenergy balance with the correcting magnets (step 2), stopping the autoimmune attack that accompanies imbalances with PMGs (step 3) and determining the correct nutrition for your body (step 4).

But knowledge alone will not restore bioenergy balance. You've got to do the things you need to do to restore bioenergy balance. The Biohealth System is not a "hit or miss" or "do it if I feel like it" thing. You can't test one day and not test again for another month and expect to restore bioenergy balance. You can't use the correcting magnet for a couple of hours and forget about using it tomorrow. You can't eat right this week and go back to another diet or not take your supplements or PMGs the next. While on the program you must continually test to be sure you are on target.

The Biohealth System must be applied with dedication and diligence.

When you remove the correcting magnet, immediately check the organ. If it checks balanced, check to see how long it remains balanced. The longer it remains balanced, the closer to healthy the organ is. When it stays balanced, the organ is healthy.

Step 6—Proving Biological Health

Proving that you have achieved biological health means two things. First, you prove that your own body can now achieve and maintain balanced bioenergy fields and keep you healthy. Second, you have removed or deactivated the causes of the problem. As long as the factors that initially caused the bioenergy imbalance are still active your body will not, without help, be able to restore and maintain bioenergy balance. As long as you have to use the magnet and PMG, causative factors are still operative and the fertile field of disease still exists.

Only when you prove that your own body, on its own, can restore and maintain bioenergy balance do you know that the original causative factors for the problem are no longer operative. Only then do you know that you've created an environment in which your body can produce health.

Proof is the essential conclusion. Believe nothing, test everything!

During the workshops I gave with Dr. Broeringmeyer, I'd often ask students at the end of the workshop, "Anyone who doesn't believe what we've said here today, please raise your hand." A very few did. Then I'd ask, "Anyone who believes what we've said today, please raise your hand." Most did.

After all raised their hands, I'd tell them, "Everyone who raised their hand has failed this course! You believe nothing, including me, until you test it."

Our purpose is not for me to tell you what is right for you. It is to give you a way to test and by this testing know what is correct for you. Below are the two methods we use in the Biohealth System for testing and proving biological health.

The test magnet tells you when you have achieved bioenergy balance. But it does not tell you if your body can maintain the balance. This is important because if your body cannot maintain the bioenergy balance, there are still causative factors you have not corrected.

There are two methods to prove your body can maintain balanced bioenergy and health. Until you prove it you do not have biohealth. Here are the two ways:

Method 1—Retracing

This is an old method based on the philosophy that to cure a disease you have to go through the steps that caused it—in reverse order.

Suppose you have an organ that tests positive to the south pole. You go through the Biohealth steps with the correcting magnet, PMGs and nutrition and finally get no response to either the north or south pole when you test the organ. The organ's bioenergetic field is now in balance. This is what you want.

But is this the result of the magnet and PMGs or is your body now producing its own balanced bioenergy and health? Do you know if the factors that originally caused the imbalance are still operative and will soon produce another imbalance? How can you know you have eliminated the field that grew the imbalance and replaced it with a field that will grow health?

After you have achieved balanced energy, you need to prove that your body is capable of producing and maintaining health by itself. This also proves that the factors that initially caused the imbalance are no longer operative.

Here is how you prove it. After you have achieved organ balance, you apply the north pole of the correcting magnet to the organ and use it until you get a north pole imbalance.

You now have a north pole imbalance. Without using correcting magnets, PMGs or anything other than nutrition, in two to four weeks your body by itself returns the imbalance to balance. This gives you proof that your body is now able to restore balance by itself and produce health. It proves you have deactivated the factors that initially produced the imbalance. It proves your body is now growing healthy!

One caution here: It's important to remember that we use the north pole to create an imbalance and prove health here. Recall our earlier discussion of disease. A north pole imbalance results in only a weak cell. The body, if functioning properly, should be able to correct this imbalance on its own and prove health.

A south pole imbalance is a more serious malfunction. The magnet and PMGs may be needed to restore balance. We don't want to make you ill. We just want to weaken the cell to make sure the body can correct it and return it to balance. That's why we use a north pole imbalance.

Method 2–The Maintenance Method

In this method, we stop the magnet and PMG when the organ returns to balanced bioenergy. We continue with the nutrition, exercise program and whatever you may have done to control stress, toxicity and other disease factors, but we do not create an imbalance as above.

Instead, every second day for the next two weeks we check the organ for balance. If it remains in balance, we then check it every week for the next month. If the organ still remains balanced, we check it every two weeks for the next two months. (If you wish to check more often, that's fine but the previous procedure should be enough.)

When, at the end of three months, the organ is still balanced you have proof your body is maintaining balance and producing Biohealth. Our preference for proving health is to use method 1 above and back it up with method 2. This will provide you with the highest degree of certainty. But the choice of methods is up to you. Either or both can do the job.

Step 7–Maintaining Correct Function

This is the final step in the Biohealth Process and is the ultimate goal of the system: After achieving health and proving it, your next goal is to keep it. Continue with your nutrition, exer-

190

cise program (the isorobic program I describe in Chapter 15 is excellent) and any successful lifestyle changes you've adopted and, above all, keep testing. Remember that, as stress and life changes occur, so do your needs change.

Testing is the key. Use your own judgment on how often to test but, above all, test. Life is a dynamic process. By continually monitoring your body for any imbalances you can keep your bioenergy fields in balance and your body functioning correctly.

Indeed, that is the whole idea behind the Biohealth System. It's not only to get you healthy. It's to keep you healthy. Believe nothing! Test everything!

In this chapter you've been given a reliable, proven, innovative system for achieving and maintaining your bioenergy balance and your health. With the Biohealth Program you determine what is best for you, what has no value for you and what is harmful to you. This gives you control over both your health and your life. If you have read this far and you are excited, I would recommend you buy the magnets and whatever else you need, read through the book, and do every step.

I'd like to end this chapter with a poem by the nineteenth-century English poet Samuel Taylor Coleridge:

What if you slept?

And what if

in your sleep

you dreamed?

And what if

in your dream

you went to heaven

and there plucked
a strange and
beautiful flower?
And what if,
when you awoke
you had that flower
in your hand?

For the biohealth student the Biohealth System is "that flower."

CHAPTER 13

Some Important Odds and Ends–Healthy Foods and Disease Patterns

*The true intention of life is happiness. We are
mad if we do not see this. We squander our
opportunity for joy.*

—Llewelyn Powys, *Impassioned Clay*

The single most important factor in achieving health is your ability to test. Since bioenergy balance produces health and bioenergy imbalance produces disease, having the ability to discover and choose what will bring you bioenergy balance and avoid those things that will destroy bioenergy balance is a very powerful thing.

The Biohealth System gives you that power through its ability to test most of what you eat and do. Knowing how to test when you have an imbalance and correct that imbalance, and then knowing how to test when you have balance and knowing how not to destroy this balance, is the foundation of the Biohealth System.

Turning Unhealthy Food Into Healthy Food

Food can really be a problem for somebody trying to maintain a health program. Even with all the testing you're going to have problems getting healthy food. Pesticides and other chemicals used to protect food and enhance its commercial value can render them virtually inedible.

Hazel Parcells found that when foods were sprayed with pesticides, it was impossible to remove the chemicals. You could wash them. You could peel them. You could cut little pieces out of the inside. Whatever you did, the chemicals remained in the food making it harmful to eat.

Obviously, you do not want to eat food that will be harmful. You would be undoing many of the positive things the Biohealth System or any health program can do for you. That's why Hazel searched out two simple ways to neutralize the chemicals in foods and make them digestible and healthy.

The first method involves Clorox. Hazel found that putting foods into a simple Clorox solution (only the original, true Clorox works) deactivated the chemicals in the foods. You use a half teaspoon of Clorox for each gallon of water and soak foods for the length of time charted below.

Type of Food	Length in Clorox Solution
Leafy vegetables	5 to 10 minutes
Root and heavy fiber vegetables	10 to 15 minutes
Medium-skinned fruits	10 minutes
Thick-skinned fruits	10 to 15 minutes
Citrus fruits	15 minutes
Bananas	30 minutes
Meat and poultry per pound	10 minutes

When the Clorox bath is completed, wash the foods in fresh water for 15 minutes. You must make a fresh bath each time you treat the foods.

Another way to remove chemicals from food involves an old friend of ours—magnets!

To magnetically treat food, use four 3,700 gauss 2 by 4 magnets (like the correcting magnets used earlier). Get a box from your grocery store that is just large enough to hold the foods you will treat. The smallest box you can get that will hold the food is best.

Place two magnets below the bottom of the box, at each side of the box, with the south poles facing up. Then place two magnets on the top of the box, at each side of the box, with the south poles facing down. With the south pole of the upper magnets facing down and the south pole of the lower magnets facing up, the entire inside of the box becomes a south pole field. Whatever you place in this box will be in a magnetic south pole field.

The food to be treated is placed in the box for 30 to 60 minutes. (Leaving it in longer does no harm, but we've found that 45 minutes in the box generally does the trick.) The magnets neutralize the chemicals and give you the same results as the Clorox bath. In the end, the food checks as clean and good as food grown organically.

Magnets may also work with people who are "allergic" to certain foods. We took a person who was allergic to tomatoes, for instance, and tested him holding the tomato. His arm dropped. When we washed the tomato and tested again, his arm still dropped. We peeled the tomato and he tested positive again. We cut little pieces out of the inside—same result.

Then we put the tomato in Clorox. His arm was strong. The same thing happened after putting the tomato in a south pole magnetic field. His allergy was not to the tomato but to the chemicals with which it had been sprayed. When the toxins and chemicals were deactivated by the Clorox or south pole magnetic field, the allergies were no longer in evidence.

You will often get a bad reading on foods before you detoxify them and a good reading following either of the treatments above.

It's important to know that the treatments above won't work 100 percent of the time. For instance, irradiated foods can't be treated this way and turned healthy. But in most cases, these treatments will work and pay big dividends in your pursuit of Biohealth. As usual, the way to know is to test!

Turning the unhealthy food you eat into healthy food is an important part of any health program. We urge you to make it a part of your life immediately and continue with it as long as you live.

Disease Patterns

Another important thing magnetic testing can do is indicate tendencies people may have toward specific diseases. Testing north or south pole on a particular group of organs can indicate a susceptibility to diseases that strike those organs and serve as a predictor of future illness.

Dr. Richard Broeringmeyer identified several of these "disease patterns" through clinical observation. In working with people who had specific diseases, Dr. Richard found that most had patterns of magnetic imbalance that made them susceptible to the disease. He also found many people who had a disease pattern but did not have the disease. Yet, in many of those cases, the disease patterns were predictive. These people were healthy at the moment but when they got under enough stress, Dr. Broeringmeyer found that the disease pattern would manifest itself and produce the disease.

Working with him, I saw many people come into workshops with these energy patterns and no disease. His response was always the same. "Wait," he'd say. "When they get under enough stress, they'll get the disease." He was right.

These disease patterns provided great knowledge and an early warning system. Unfortunately, sometimes people had a hard time coming to grips with what Dr. Broeringmeyer was saying. It was hard for them to realize that they were susceptible to a disease until they actually got the disease.

I remember one workshop where a woman got up in front of the group and announced that Dr. Broeringmeyer was crazy after he told her she had a diabetic energy pattern. She told him she had no symptoms of diabetes and that what he was saying was total nonsense. Then she stormed from the room. We didn't see her again until two years later when she came to a course we were giving to apologize to Dr. Broeringmeyer. She announced that after experiencing a period of stress, she was now taking insulin for her diabetes. He had been correct.

These patterns are not cast in bronze, of course. Nothing we tell you is. You are not a statistic. You are a unique individual. These patterns are a guide. They have to be applied to your own, unique existence. Discovery of the patterns is merely a device for waking you up and reminding you that, if you're in a pattern like this, you need to do something about it.

Knowledge of these patterns has been very valuable in helping many people. It showed them where to look for possible problems. And, of equal importance, it led them to an understanding of the most important fact about disease: When you correct destructive energy patterns, you no longer have disease. Discovering these patterns and using the Biohealth System take you back to a place medical science often bypasses—the source of the disease.

For any health problem, you must first discover the energy pattern that is producing the problem. Second, you correct and balance those energy patterns that are causing the problem. Doing this changes the environment—the soil of the body—from one that grows malfunction and disease to one that grows balanced function and health. That, in a nutshell, is what the Biohealth System does.

The following is a list of disease patterns identified by Dr. Broeringmeyer. What is important is that if you have a pattern you take action to correct it. "Hypo" means you get a north pole reading on the organ. "Hyper" means you get a south pole reading.

- Alcoholism—The energy pattern for alcoholism includes hypo-adrenals, hypo-liver, hypo-kidney, hypo-pituitary and hypo-spleen. The north pole adrenals (hypo-adrenals) must be present. When you combine hypo-adrenals with any three of the other four indicators, you have the disease pattern for alcoholism. For instance, hypo-adrenals with hypo-kidney, hypo-liver and hypo-spleen would indicate an alcoholism disease pattern. To avoid the possibility of alcoholism, you would balance bioenergy for each of these organs.

- Allergy—The energy pattern indicators for allergies include hypo-pancreas, hypo-liver, hypo-colon, hypo-adrenals, hyper-kidney and hypo-pituitary. Hyper-kidney and hypo-colon are the key indicators here. When you combine them with any other two indicators you have an energy pattern for allergy.

- Anemia—Energy pattern indicators include hypo-liver, hypo-stomach, hyper-adrenals, hypo-colon and hypo-thyroid. Hypo-liver, hypo-stomach and hyper-adrenals are required for the anemia energy pattern. The other two indicators may or may not be present but usually are.

- Bowel disorders—Indicators include hypo-colon and hyper-colon. Either one or both indicate the energy pattern for the problem.

- Diabetes mellitus—Indicators include hypo-liver and/or hypo-gall bladder, hypo-pancreas and hyper-adrenals. These three indicate the disease pattern of diabetes mellitus. Add to these hyper-pituitary and you could have a diabetes insipidus pattern.

- Epilepsy—Indicators include hypo-kidneys, hypo-adrenals, hypo-colon, hypo-stomach, hyper-stomach and hyper-pancreas. Hypo-kidneys, hypo-adrenals and hypo-colon form the basis of the pattern. Any one or all three of the other indicators may also be present.

- High blood pressure/Hypertension—Indicators include hyper or hypo-kidneys, hyper-adrenals, hypo-liver, hypo-pancreas, hypo-spleen and hypo-colon. The kidney and hyper-adrenal imbalances must be present for this energy pattern. Any of the other three may be present. Usually all three are present.

- Low blood pressure/Hypotension—Indicators include hypo-left ventricle of the heart, hypo-liver, hyper-pancreas, hyper-spleen, hypo-adrenals, hypo-colon, hypo-pituitary and hyper or hypo-kidneys. The heart, liver and adrenal readings are necessary for this pattern. Any of the others may also be present.

- Sinusitis—Indicators include hyper-kidneys, hypo-colon and hyper-lungs. The kidney reading is required for the sinusitis energy pattern. Any or both of the others may also be present.

Dr. Broeringmeyer found stress plays a major role when these disease patterns ultimately produced disease. An imbalanced adrenal gland is strongly associated with stress. Not surprisingly, an imbalanced adrenal gland is present in all but two of the disease patterns.

These patterns are entirely the work of Dr. Broeringmeyer and I thank him for them. Although not 100 percent predictive, the existence of these patterns should be taken seriously and serve as a motivator for monitoring and using preventive measures.

Some Biohealth Reminders

Step 1—Testing

- When first learning test areas, use diagrams and locate the areas on your body

- Tell the subject to resist before applying pressure

- Use surrogate or other test when arms are too strong or weak

- Do not use magnets on pregnant women or those with pace-maker/implanted medical devices

Step 2—Restoring Energy Balance

- Use the pole that is the opposite to the pole that caused the arm to go weak

- Use the same pole to face the organ being tested for both the correcting and the holding magnets

- If you use the more convenient super magnet, excluding cancer and infections, switch to the 2 by 4 magnet if results aren't satisfactory

- Wear a thin garment between the skin and magnet to avoid skin irritation

- Do the five majors first (except with infections and cancer)

- If colon imbalanced, correct it along with the five majors

- Always use north pole of the 2 by 4 magnet on cancer and infection

Step 3–Stopping the Autoimmune Attack

- Use the PMG routinely

- Continue to use the PMG as long as you continue with the magnet

- PMGs often can't be tested. But if you use a correcting magnet you use a PMG

Step 4–Determining the Correct Nutrition for You

- Use the test magnet to determine what your body is telling you it needs

- Test for both quality and quantity; if your arm gets strong on two or more readings, use the larger amount to correct more severe problems and the smaller amount for minor problems and for health maintenance

- Use the same supplement for more than one area, when possible

- The Standard Process test kit and others like it can be very valuable and time saving

Step 5–Applying and Monitoring the Program

- Dedication and commitment are essential
- Test, test and test again
- Only by continual monitoring can you be sure you are on target
- Monitor until you have achieved balanced bioenergy, then prove it

Step 6–Proving the Program

- Create a north pole imbalance in the organ being tested
- Have your own body return the imbalance to balance without magnets or PMGs
- When your own body corrects the north pole imbalance you have biohealth

Step 7–Maintaining Health and Function

- Life is dynamic
- The best way to fight disease is to never get any
- The goal is not to get healthy but to stay healthy
- This can be done with continual monitoring

CHAPTER 14

Three Deadly Problems–Cancer, Heart Disease and Pain

Life is deeper than we could have imagined, more unscrupulous, more vigorous, more exultant.

—Llewelyn Powys, *The Cradle of God*

This chapter is based on clinical experience. In it, we will give you information on Biohealth approaches to three serious problems—cancer, heart disease and pain. These are not treatment recommendations nor do they replace treatment or the need for a health professional. They are offered purely as information that, after you validate it or invalidate it with your testing, may be of value to you.

Whatever your present approach to these problems, or whatever you may decide to do in relation to them, this information could be of help to you. Should you choose to test it and find it useful, you may want to work it into your program. It's been a great help for many people but, in the final analysis, you and your health professional will have to make the final decision.

Cancer and Bioelectromagnetics

The following information is based primarily on the clinical work of Dr. Broeringmeyer. In the workshops Dr. Broeringmeyer and I collaborated on we saw many cancer patients and had many successes. I saw the program we outline in this chapter work on hundreds of people, including myself.

After we'd teach our students the Biohealth System and the additional cancer regimen included in this chapter, many came back as quickly as six months later cancer free! We had many inspiring successes. Regrettably, we also had failures. I'll do my best to describe both and the reasons for them in this chapter.

First, it is important to say that we did not "treat" the people. We gave them advice and guidance in the course of our workshops. As with all things in the Biohealth System, the emphasis was on the person himself and his ability to do the things necessary to attain and maintain Biohealth. We teach how to do testing that may be of great value.

Second, it must be pointed out that research measuring the effects of magnets on cancer has been done on animals and plants but, to the best of my knowledge, no research on humans has been financed or done. There are some excellent writings on cancer and bioelectromagnetics in books by Albert Roy Davis, Walter Rawls and Dr. Robert Becker (see the reading list at the end of this book) and we recommend them highly but human research has not yet been done.

This is why the clinical observations of Dr. Broeringmeyer are so important. We offer them not as a treatment program but as something that you may test and use as you and your health practitioner see fit.

North Pole Magnetic Energy and Cancer

The first requirement in an anti-cancer program is to stop the growth of the cancer. Cancer is very acid and, therefore, strongly south pole. Research by Nobel Prize winner Otto

Warburg and others has shown that cancer cells grow with very little oxygen and thus do not efficiently produce energy. Cancer cells metabolize glucose into lactic acid, which is one reason why cancer cells are so acid and south pole. It also tells us that cancer cells do not grow and survive in a high oxygen environment.

In addition, it was found that cancer cells do not reproduce or grow in an alkaline environment. When placed in an alkaline medium with a pH of 7.6 they stop multiplying. At a pH of 8.2 to 8.5 the life cycle of the cancer cell stops entirely and in a few hours it dies. According to this research it's obvious that, to stop cancer cells from growing, we want two things: an alkaline environment and oxygen.

What, when applied to any cell, increases the alkalinity within the cell and brings in more oxygen? The magnetic north pole! As discussed earlier, the north pole removes hydrogen ions, which increases alkalinity while increasing oxygen in the area it effects.

The test magnet tells us the location of the cancer and where to apply the north pole, and we do this immediately. However, *the test magnet does not diagnose cancer.* Cancer is diagnosed by a biopsy. The people Dr. Broeringmeyer and I saw all had a biopsy that diagnosed the cancer. We insisted on it. The test magnet is used to determine where to place the north pole to stop the cancer growth and monitor our progress—not to diagnose it.

Both the correcting magnet and super magnet have been used for cancer. However, two 3,700 gauss magnets penetrate deeper and cover a larger area than the smaller 12,500 gauss super magnet. Since cancers often cover a larger area and require deep penetration, we prefer the two 2 by 4 magnets for cancer.

Always, as soon as possible and as much as possible, you use the north pole on any cancer. It will turn the inside of the cells alkaline and increase the amount of oxygen in the area. This slows down cancer growth while avoiding negative effects on normal cells. Also, along with the magnet, you should immediately start to use the correct PMG to negate the effects of any autoimmune attack.

The goal of the Biohealth System is not to kill or treat the cancer cells, but to replace the cancer cells with healthy cells. The following outlines the Biohealth Program for achieving this goal.

Protomophogen

Where available, PMGs must be used to stop the autoimmune attack on the cancerous organ.

Minerals and Cancer:
The Phospholipid Wrapping

What follows is an oversimplified presentation of a complex subject that will provide both accurate and crucial information.

Specific minerals are formed in every cell and, ultimately, these minerals control the division of the cell. It is their job to see that cell division is controlled. Obviously, in cancer, cell division is uncontrolled.

Research done by Brasilford Robertson, Fenton Turck and Royal Lee found that these minerals are covered by a phospholipid wrapping, or a wrapping of fat. As long as this wrapping stayed in place, cell division was controlled. Cancer does not occur. But when the phospholipid wrapping is removed, uncontrolled cell division could occur. Many carcinogens remove this phospholipid wrapping. When that happens, cell division becomes uncontrolled, which leads to cancer.

In cancer, routinely, no phospholipid wrapping was found on the minerals in this research. It was concluded that, in cancer, restoring the phospholipid wrapping is very important (see Royal Lee's book, *Protomorphology*).

To restore that wrapping, Lee devised a supplement called Super EFF. It is a Standard Process supplement. Six to nine capsules are taken on an empty stomach every day. Two to three tablespoons of flax seed may also be used. All of the people we worked with who had cancer used Super EFF because it is the most efficient way known to restore the phospholipid wrapping to the minerals.

Cancer and Two Homeopathic Remedies

Jack Schwarz, one of my greatest teachers, found two homeopathic remedies that directly related to cancer cells. We won't discuss homeopathy in this book but we will pass along the homeopathics identified by Jack that we have our people with cancer use.

The substances are viscum album (mistletoe) and vitis vinifera (European grape juice). Mistletoe has been used in the treatment of cancer since 1920. These homeopathics come in a 60 ml bottle with a dropper. The strength of the homeopathic remedy used is 1D and you take 20 drops at a time. The 20 drops are placed under the tongue and taken when a person wakes up in the morning and before they go to sleep.

The person with cancer orders these two substances and takes them as directed until he or she has proven there is no more cancer.

In the appendix, you'll find information on where to obtain these substances.

Cancer and Pancreatic Enzymes, and the Pancreas

Another important area for cancer care is pancreatic enzymes. In almost all cancer patients, the pancreas is not working correctly. Pancreatic enzymes play an important role in the digestion of food. With the pancreas malfunctioning, digestion is poor.

Cancer cells also build a form of shielding that protects them from immune system cells. Pancreatic enzymes remove these shields so immune cells can get through to attack the cancer cells.

There are many good sources for pancreatic enzymes. I use Pan 10X which you can purchase from Nu Biologics (information in the index to this book). Use the test magnet to determine how many capsules to take with each meal.

I also recommend taking an additional eight capsules of Pan 10X on an empty stomach preferably two or three times a day. The capsules taken with meals help to digest food. The capsules taken on an empty stomach help digest the cancer cells and their protective covering.

Once the cancer area is retraced and health is proven, the person can stop using the pancreatic enzymes. We recommend continuing them until you return to a normal pancreatic reading and prove you no longer have cancer.

In almost all cancers, the pancreas and kidneys are malfunctioning. We recommend returning the kidneys and pancreas to balanced energy.

Cancer and the Liver

The liver is a special problem. A major food for cancer cells is glucose. The liver produces glucose which helps feed the cancer cells. Therefore it helps to minimize the amount of glucose the liver produces.

A south pole liver produces the most glucose. Therefore, immediately, with a south pole liver you use the north pole correcting magnet and the liver PMG.

To produce the least glucose we would like a north pole liver. Whether we will keep a north pole liver depends on the kidneys. The liver and kidneys are a team. To replace cancer you must have a balanced kidney.

As long as the kidney is not balanced, our aim is to balance the liver. When the kidney is balanced, and for as long as it is balanced, we prefer a north pole liver.

Cancer and the Thymus

Stimulating your own body to remove cancer—or prevent it—is one of the most powerful tools available to you. Your immune system is designed to remove things from your body that shouldn't be there—such as cancer cells—and replace them with what should be there—healthy cells.

A very important and powerful part of the immune system that accomplishes this are the T cells. T cells are a type of white blood cell that destroys foreign substances like cancer cells and bacteria. T cells are manufactured in your thymus gland. By stimulating your thymus gland, your body produces more of the T cells that will remove your cancer cells.

A very effective method for stimulating the thymus gland is the use of the south pole of the super magnet on the thymus. The super magnet has a very high gauss of 12,500 and has proved excellent at producing the desired effect on the thymus.

To stimulate the thymus gland, place the south pole of the super magnet over the gland. Initially, when you check your thymus with the test magnet, it may read north pole or neutral. Keep the super magnet on the thymus until it reads south pole. At that point, you know you are stimulating the thymus.

Even when the thymus is reading south pole we have you continue to stimulate it with the super magnet. It is that important to keep the thymus functioning south pole. You continue using the super magnet south pole so every time you take a test magnet reading of your thymus gland it will be south pole.

And here's a good side effect from stimulating the thymus: There is evidence that thymic hormones retard the aging process. When you stimulate your thymus gland, it will produce more of these anti-aging hormones.

To further stimulate the thymus gland we also use the Standard Process foods that stimulate it. Use the Thymus PMG, of course, and Thymex. To help stimulate the entire immune system, also use Immuplex.

Cancer and the Spleen

The spleen is an important organ in the immune system. Therefore it is very important to balance it. To balance the spleen use the correcting magnet, the spleen PMG, and the spleen nutrition. As soon as possible, balance the spleen.

Cancer and the Thyroid Gland

Almost all people with cancer are also hypothyroid. Their thyroid gland is functioning slowly as is their metabolism. During his work, Dr. Broeringmeyer studied a group of people who were healthy and found that the one thing they all had in common was that they were slightly hyperthyroid. In other words, the thyroid was slightly overactive.

Research at Sloan-Kettering Hospital showed that while it was easy to transplant a cancer into a hypothyroid animal, it was not possible to transplant cancer into a slightly hyperthyroid animal. The cancer wouldn't survive. It must be only slightly hyperactive, because when the thyroid gland becomes highly overactive, it becomes thyrotoxic and that is as bad as being hypothyroid.

That's why the slightly hyperthyroid gland is the best. To avoid all diseases, and especially avoid or stop cancer, you want a slightly hyperthyroid gland.

How do you know when your thyroid is slightly overactive? By far the best way we know is with the magnet.

When you get a south pole reading on your thyroid and all five majors are normal, you have a slightly hyperthyroid gland. This is what we want to achieve for all people with cancer people—and for everyone.

If you get a south pole reading on your thyroid and any of the five majors are unbalanced, you probably are excessively hyperthyroid and thyrotoxic. Our objective is to have you return all five majors to balance and then have a south pole thyroid.

Based on the work of Dr. Broeringmeyer, as long as you are slightly hyperthyroid you have great resistance to disease.

Cancer and Tuberculinum 100C

Hazel Parcells had much success with cancer and on every cancer, regardless of where it was or what kind it was, she used the homeopathic Tuberculinum 100C (the "100C" indicates the strength of the dosage and how it is energized or percussed).

Tuberculinum 100C comes in the form of granules. You take four granules four times a day. The granules are held under the tongue and allowed to dissolve there. Clinically, they have been shown to be a big help in the fight against cancer.

Cancer and Mycosurge

Mycosurge is a German remedy that consists of 12 mushrooms. It is available in the U.S. from Marco Pharma. Mycosurge has mushrooms in it that stimulate the immune system and have strong anti-tumor activity.

You cannot buy direct from Marco Pharma, but you can buy it from a health professional that deals with Marco Pharma.

Cancer and MGN3 and CO Q10

We have recently had some good testing and good results with MGN3 and CO Q10. I would recommend testing them. They are available from many sources, one of which is Nu Biologics.

Cancer Metabolism

One of the great, inspired discoveries of our time came through the work of Dr. Otto Warburg. Dr. Warburg was awarded the Nobel Prize for his discovery that a major difference between normal cells and cancer cells was the fact that normal cells use oxygen for energy production while cancer cells don't.

The cancer cell and normal cell thus use different methods to produce their energy.

Both the cancer cell and normal cell begin by using glucose as the raw material for energy production but there the resemblance ends. The normal cell combines oxygen with glucose and yields 40 energy units for each molecule of glucose used. The cancer cell breaks down glucose without oxygen and yields only 2 energy units per molecule of glucose.

Healthy cells give energy to the body but cancer cells remove energy from the body. The anaerobic (without oxygen) breakdown of glucose in cancer cells produces a large amount of lactic acid. However, since the yield of energy from glucose is so low in the cancer cell, the cancer cell has an enormous appetite for glucose. To maintain its energy it wants more and more glucose. The liver, and to some extent, the kidney will convert some lactic acid back into glucose again. With the cancer cell's enormous appetite, the liver and kidneys are stimulated to produce this glucose from the lactic acid waste of cancer metabolism.

This is where things really get sticky. The production of one molecule of glucose from lactic acid requires at least 6 energy units. As a result, for every molecule of glucose made for the cancer cell 6 units of energy are taken from the body and only 2 units are given back.

Thus, cancer takes a great deal of energy from the body. Dr. Broeringmeyer found that when the cancer took 35 percent of the body's total energy, the heart would stop beating.

With this in mind, the impetus for immediately instituting the Biohealth cancer program becomes even more urgent.

Cancer and Healthy Food

Without going into detail, many raw vegetables and fruits have been shown to have phytochemicals (plant chemicals) that fight cancer. Whole food supplements with cancer fighting phytochemicals are becoming available. Decontaminate them with Clorox or magnets. Avoid refined carbohydrates and processed foods.

Standard Process makes such a whole food called Phytolyn, which consists of kale and Brussels sprouts. Their phytochemicals fight cancer and are particularly effective against carcinogens.

Monitoring Cancer

How can you know—not hope or guess—that you are slowing down your cancer? There are two very simple ways.

The first involves Biological Terrain Assessment (BTA). We'll discuss this more fully in the next chapter but, for now, we'll give you information on how to use one of its readings to confirm your success in treating cancer. The reading we're interested in here is of the *oxidation reduction* (redox) potential of the blood given by the BTA instrument. Research initially in France and Germany, and now in the United States, has shown a high correlation between blood redox levels and cancer. Cancer closely correlates to a high redox reading. A normal redox reading correlates with an environment in which cancer cannot grow. Every cancer we have seen has had a high redox reading.

When the blood redox reading goes from a high cancer reading to a normal reading, the body has created an environment in which it is very difficult, if not impossible, for cancer cells to live. With the Biohealth Program (or any program), when the BTA redox reading goes from the high range (in which cancer grows) to the health range (in which cancer does not grow) the cancer generally can no longer be found. As a result, Biohealth where available uses the BTA redox reading to monitor the progress of the program.

A second way to monitor progress is through liver and kidney testing with your test magnet. Almost invariably, the liver and kidneys will have an unbalanced reading with cancer. Keep checking the kidneys for a balanced reading. Getting a balanced reading with the kidneys, even though the cancer is still reading south pole, indicates that your treatment may be succeeding.

Many times you can not balance the kidneys until you balance the liver.

Obviously, the very best reading of all is when the south pole reading of the cancerous organ returns to normal.

Our Failures–Why?

Yes, we had failures. Why?

There were two major conditions that spelled failure. First, and most common, was failure of the kidneys to respond. No matter what was done, they didn't improve. In fact, they usually got worse. When that happened, the person's cancer usually got worse. That is why, in addition to the cancer program we evaluate the pancreas and kidneys—especially the kidneys. Unless the kidney can be balanced the person often doesn't make it.

The second condition that spelled failure was stress. If stress cannot be brought under control, it can be a killer. Where the history of a person indicated stress, we almost always found the adrenals unbalanced. In this situation we paid special attention to training people to check their adrenals at home. We were sure to tell them that, unless they could get the stress in their life under control, it would be difficult to heal.

We found the test magnet to be very helpful here. Having information about bioenergy balance in the adrenal glands lets people know that they are having trouble with stress and when they need to do something about it. We taught them to monitor their response to stress by monitoring the adrenals and, often, we found them better able to deal with it, especially when using the stress control techniques we gave them.

For the stressed person it is important to balance the liver, kidneys and adrenals.

Heart Disease

Heart disease is the biggest killer in our country today. It can come quickly and tragically with little, if any, warning. Dr. Royal

Lee was the first to recognize that *sudden death from heart attack was essentially the product of a B complex and E complex vitamin deficiency disease syndrome.* I emphasize this not only because of its overall importance, but also because so little attention is paid to it. When you understand the importance of it, it will go a long way toward helping you prevent heart disease.

Remember, we do not diagnose or fight disease. Fighting disease does not cause health. Health removes disease and produces an immunity to disease. The aim of the Biohealth System is to cause health. So, to prevent heart attacks, you have to know what causes a healthy heart.

What causes a healthy heart? To answer this, you need to answer only one associated question: What causes your heart to beat?

A flow of electricity causes your heart to beat. Approximately 72 times per minute your heart gets an electric shock, an electrical stimulation, and 72 times per minute it beats. A diseased heart does not beat correctly. A fatal heart attack occurs when the heart stops beating. To create a healthy heart we have to know what produces the electric current that keeps it beating.

Surprisingly, we have known what this is since 1935.

The Research

The discovery of what makes a heart beat and keeps it beating was made by a pigeon raiser in England named Carter. Some of his pigeons developed paralyzed wings. He found this was due to defective transmission of electrical impulses. Carter found that the pigeons were completely cured when he fed them whole wheat.

But Carter wasn't satisfied with this simple explanation. He wondered what caused this to happen. He found that when he fed his pigeons the fat-soluble B vitamins, there was no improvement in their condition. He concluded that there must be something in the whole wheat we didn't know existed that was curing the heart block.

Carter was able to isolate the factors in B complex vitamins and discovered a B_4 vitamin. Later, we found that B_1 and B_4 vitamins occur together in nature but nobody seemed to be aware of the existence of B_4 at the time. Carter found a way to remove the B_4 factor for experimental purposes and experienced some stunning results.

Whenever he gave his pigeons food deficient in B_4, their wings would become paralyzed. When he gave them B_4, the paralysis disappeared.

Carter published his findings in 1935 but little attention was paid to it. Today we know that B_4 is the nerve motor conducting factor of the nervous system. And of the heart. Without B_4, the electric current needed for correct heart function is not adequate.

B_4 and B_1

At first glance, it might appear that there wasn't a problem here. With B_4 occurring with B_1 in nature, you'd think there couldn't be a shortage. And there might not be, except for the law and processed foods.

B_4 has been shown to be safe and necessary for nerve conduction in pigeons and other animals but not human beings. So, by law, it can't be added to human food. Nor can it appear in any supplements.

In the processing of many foods the B vitamins are removed and later restored. The problem is that they are restored without the B_4, since it hasn't been approved as safe and necessary for human beings. B_4 can't be added so the processed foods go without B_4.

Fortunately, when you find supplements made from whole foods like the Standard Process supplements, you get an answer for this problem. Standard Process makes a supplement called Cataplex B. This is a natural whole food that has in it the entire B complex, including B_4.

In the whole natural unprocessed food if you have B_1, you have B_4. Likewise, in supplements made of whole unprocessed food when you have B_1, you have B_4. That is why whole foods are such a necessity and processed foods such a problem. We do not even have knowledge of all the phytochemicals in plants. The only way to be sure you get the whole complex, including the B_4, is to use whole foods.

Thanks to the genius of Dr. Royal Lee, the Standard Process products are all whole foods. Cataplex B has in it B_1 and B_4. The B_4 is not added. It is a natural part of the whole food complex from which Standard Process Cataplex B is made.

Cataplex is the name the Standard Process people use for a whole food product. When you see this name, you know you are getting a whole food product. As a result, when a person takes Cataplex B they know they are getting all the B vitamins including B_4.

Below, we list, in sequence, some symptoms of heart disease that could lead to a heart attack. These are warning signals for heart disease and a possible heart attack. B_4 plays a big role in each.

You don't need to have any or all of these symptoms for a heart attack, of course. Sometimes heart attacks occur without symptoms or warning signals. But by learning about the cause of these symptoms, you will understand what makes your heart beat and what you need to do to keep it beating.

As usual, this is not medical advice, nor is it a substitute for medical diagnosis and treatment. It is information you can test that may be of help to you.

Arrhythmia

A first sign of heart malfunction is arrhythmia. Arrythmia simply means a lack of consistent rhythm in the beating of the heart. Lacking B_4 at times there will not be sufficient nerve electric current in the heart to keep it beating regularly. It has been found in many clinical reports that if a person with arrhythmia is given Cataplex B to chew, a regular rhythm will return to the heart in as little time as 10 minutes.

Heart Murmurs

These are also called "regurgitating" murmurs. Because of a lack of nerve current, the heart valve does not shut completely when it beats. It only closes 99 percent, so the blood goes back through that slight opening and makes a sound.

The disease beriberi is listed in medical literature as being caused by a lack of thiamine (vitamin B_1). Among the many symptoms of beriberi is heart murmur. However, where there is a lack of B_1 there must also be a lack of B_4 since they occur together. While lack of B_1 has been blamed for this murmur, we believe the actual cause to be B_4.

By attaching a person to an EKG or a phonocardiograph, it has been found that the heart often returns to correct function within 10 minutes of chewing Cataplex B with its B_4. If it doesn't, it usually returns within a few days.

If the murmur continues after taking Cataplex B, the person almost always had rheumatic fever as a child, a condition which scars the heart valve. Scar tissue does not conduct nerve current properly.

Heart Enlargement

Heart enlargement is a serious condition that can lead to necrosis (death or decay of heart tissue) and loss of life.

How does the heart enlarge? The truth is that it doesn't enlarge, it sags. It begins to stretch. When the heart sags it drops down in the chest, simply obeying gravity. This is a dangerous situation.

The heart sags because the muscles have lost their tone. Why do heart muscles lose tone? Because they have lost electricity. When the heart is electrically starved, it begins to stretch and sag. When it sags, the valves no longer fit. They no longer close properly because they have been stretched.

Is an enlarged heart a cause of heart disease? No. It is a symptom of lack of electricity, which is a symptom of vitamin B_4 deficiency.

218

There is a great deal more about heart irregularities that we could discuss such as fibrillation, bradycardia and extra heart beats but this would be repetitious. In general, the heart beats because of a nerve signal, which is basically an electric current that comes down a big bundle of nerve ganglia called the *bundle of His*. These nerve ganglia act like a big bundle of wires moving down the heart. The signal goes to the sinoatrial node (SA node) and atrioventricular node (AV node). These nodes then boost the electrical signal all the way to the myocardium, which is the heart muscle.

The nerve signal hits the myocardium and branches out simultaneously to the left and right ventricles of the heart. This is quite a big shock of electricity and is what makes the heart beat.

Heart disease occurs when something interferes with that electric current or nerve signal. A fatal heart attack occurs when something shuts off that current.

A major factor in keeping the electric current flowing and the heart beating is the B vitamin complex, with B_4 an essential part of it. The importance of this cannot be overestimated. Understanding and acting on it can save lives.

Vitamin E_2 and Fatal "Heart Attacks"

The importance of vitamin E to the heart was first shown in tests done by veterinarians at the University of Wisconsin in the 1940s. They removed vitamin E from the rations of cattle. Cattle do not have heart attacks—at least not until the vitamin E is taken from their rations. Within three months to two years, every head of cattle died of a heart attack.

Vitamin E increases the oxygen efficiency of the blood by *250 percent*. A specific part of the total package that makes up natural vitamin E is vitamin E_2. Vitamin E_2 rations the oxygen that is sent to the muscles.

When you exercise, the muscles seize a great deal of oxygen. If they take too much, there is not enough left for the heart. It stops beating. Vitamin E_2 rations the oxygen to the muscles and sees to it that the heart muscle receives enough oxygen.

Vitamin E_2 is the most fat soluble factor in vitamin E. It is the most easily removed factor in the refining of wheat. Synthetic vitamin E does not have vitamin E_2. Taking a synthetic vitamin E can lead to a lack of E_2.

With heart disease and a lack of vitamin E_2, exercise can lead to a fatal heart attack. During the winter people often have fatal heart attacks while shoveling snow, for instance. We are told these attacks were caused by exercising with a bad heart. But were they really? The fact is that these people don't die from shoveling snow. They die because, while shoveling snow, the muscles take up so much oxygen that not enough is left for the heart. More correctly, these people die from lack of oxygen because of a lack of vitamin E_2.

For a healthy heart, a person needs the entire vitamin E complex and most importantly, they need E_2. Standard Process makes a vitamin E_2 supplement. We recommend that all people who have heart problems and do any physical work take E_2. Any person with cardiac problems can take it.

In addition to helping the heart, E_2 is also excellent for helping to prevent muscle cramps. Many mountain climbers rely of E_2 to ration their blood oxygen and prevent cramps.

Homocysteine

There's been a lot of talk about the danger of elevated cholesterol but many people with heart disease—more than 12 million of them—have normal cholesterol. Research on homocysteine, an amino acid, helps to explain this.

Homocysteine only appears for transient periods of time during the breakdown of other proteins in the body. It appears as a result of the body's inability to break down amino acid complexes completely, which leaves homocysteine stranded in the bloodstream.

Why is this important? Because a measure of 12 percent above the normal homocysteine range yields a 340 percent increase in the risk of myocardial infarction (heart attack).

What can you do to prevent excess homocysteine? The Standard Process supplements Cataplex G and Folic Acid B$_{12}$ complete the breakdown of amino acids and prevent the production of homocysteine.

Ionizable Calcium

When your doctor listens to your heart with a stethoscope, he or she first hears a "lub" sound followed by a "dub." The "lub" is caused by the closing of the tricuspid and mitral valves, the "dub" by the closing of the semilunar valves just as the heart begins to relax. When the heart is starved of ionizable calcium, there is a "lub" there but no "dub." You usually find this "dubless" person very fatigued by the end of the day.

To rapidly restore the "dub" we have the person take ionizable calcium. Standard Process's Cataplex F restores heart sounds and increases energy. Cataplex F immediately ionizes the calcium already in your blood. When the calcium is ionized it flows into the tissues where it is needed, including the heart. Often, within minutes, the "dub" returns to the heartbeat.

A form of calcium that is rapidly ionized is calcium lactate. Usually within 24 hours after taking calcium lactate and Cataplex F the "dub" will be back and at the end of the day the person will not be so tired.

Cataplex G, C and E

These Cataplex supplements can be important to heart health and maintenance. Cataplex E and Cataplex C help the heart to repair itself. Cataplex C also increases the oxygen carrying capacity of the blood thus allowing more oxygen to get to the heart and other muscles of the body. Cataplex G produces vasodilation (opening of the blood vessels) so they don't get too

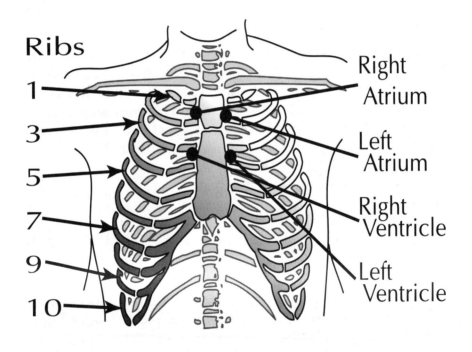

The four areas for testing the balance of the heart, and then correcting the balance of the heart.

narrow and cause possible heart disorders. It also increases blood flow and helps keep homocysteine low.

The Total Heart Program

As discussed earlier, the first step in any Biohealth Program is to evaluate and then balance energy fields. The heart is one of the five majors we discussed earlier and should be balanced before organs outside the five majors are balanced, except in cases of infection and cancer.

The heart has four chambers. Two are upper chambers (the right and left atria). Two are lower chambers (the right and left ventricles). The testing and balancing points for the hearts are actually the valves of the four chambers. All four are tested. If any are out of balance, the first thing you should do is bring them into balance.

The measurement areas for the heart are at the side of the sternum. The atria are measured between ribs one and two. The ventricles are measured between ribs three and four.

These four areas are evaluated first with the test magnet. The balancing magnet will help correct heart chambers that are out of balance. But for the heart we have a unique supplement.

Special for the heart Standard Process has developed a whole food complex called Cardio-Plus that will provide special help for people who have heart problems with high blood pressure. It contains Cardiotrophin PMG, the heart PMG. It also contains Cataplex C, E, E_2 and G along with Riboflavin, Selenium, Niacin, vitamin B_6 and Coenzyme Q10.

If a person has low blood pressure, use Vasculin instead of Cardio-Plus. With low blood pressure, the person should also use Cataplex F and D.

To balance the heart we recommend Cardio-Plus, Cataplex B and Folic Acid B_{12}. A regimen of eight to 12 Cardio-Plus, six Cataplex B and six Folic Acid B_{12} per day has frequently proven correct.

When the heart becomes balanced again, we recommend three Cardio-Plus, three Cataplex B and three Folic Acid B$_{12}$ per day for maintenance. Since the heart is in balance, you will not get any readings with the test magnet. There will be no north or south pole responses. You will know that your heart is doing fine when you continue to check your heart and get no readings with your test magnet.

Use Other Health Professionals

Obviously, with cancer and heart disease, you will need professional help. We are not telling you that the information we give you is complete. *We do not recommend "do-it-yourself" treatment of disease, especially with these two killer diseases.* Dr. Broeringmeyer and I always worked with the health professionals of our students, providing a team approach to health.

Our purpose in this book is to educate not to treat. There is no more exciting adventure on earth than knowing and exploring your own body. With our help and guidance, you've gained some expertise in the biology and physiology of your own body. You've learned much about the way your body works. When you incorporate the Biohealth System into your life and experience what it's like to bring your own body back into bioenergy balance, you'll get a doctorate in self-knowledge.

The Pain Problem

As you can tell from the quotations from Llewelyn Powys I've included in this book, I believe joy and happiness to be an important part of life. Pain and happiness are mutually exclusive. Therefore, to help restore joy to life, we must control pain.

When the cause of pain is known and can be removed, pain is not a problem. When the cause of pain is not known or can't be removed, the person has chronic pain. Magnetic energy can very often be a great help in this situation.

How and When to Use the Magnetic North Pole for Pain

Pain receptors are called *nociceptors*. Unlike other sensory receptors, pain receptors do not adapt. They continue to cause pain over time and often get worse.

Magnets often help because the surface of each nerve cell carries a positive electrical charge (the inside of the cell has a negative charge). In the case of pain, the outside positive charge increases and becomes stronger. This positive electric current produces pain. For this reason, most pain will check south pole with your test magnet. When the painful site gives a south pole reading, usually a north magnetic pole will lessen or stop the pain. The first step in pain control is seeing if there is a south pole reading where the pain is. If there is, you apply the north magnetic pole.

We don't use the correcting magnet here but a "pain magnet," which is different from the balancing magnet. Designed by Dr. Broeringmeyer, the pain magnet is more a therapy pad. It comes in a 9-inch by 12-inch sheet of 150 gauss strength. You cut the pads to the size you want and two thicknesses are placed over the painful area with the north poles facing the painful These pads can be purchased from The Cutting Edge.

Some painful areas do not give a south pole reading and are still helped by the north pole. This is especially true for back pain related to disc problems. Try the north pole over these areas and you will often get relief. There is no limit to how long the magnets can be left in place. They have no side effects.

Remember, though, magnets are not recommended for pregnant women and people wearing pacemakers or other implanted medical devices.

What If the Painful Area Is Swollen and Has Fluid?

The north pole of a magnet attracts fluid. Therefore, if an area is swollen with fluid and a north pole is placed over it, it will draw more fluid into the area and increase the pain. *A north pole is never put over an area that is swollen and fluid filled.*

With a swollen area, the magnet must first be used to remove the fluid. This will lessen the pain. There are two ways magnets can be used to remove the excess fluid. The north pole will draw fluid to it. The south pole disperses it.

To use the north pole, place the north pole about 1 to 2 inches from the fluid. The north pole will pull the fluid toward itself and out of the swollen area. To use the south pole, place the south pole directly over the area of fluid. It will disperse it. Use the south pole even if there is a south pole reading. Then, when the fluid is dispersed, immediately go to the north pole.

The Biomagnetic Therapy Pad– Using North and South Poles

There are pain conditions that do not respond to north pole energy. An example is sciatica. Sciatica develops from two conditions. The first involves inflammation of the nerve (this inflammation runs the length of the nerve). The other involves a weak muscle creating irritation in the area. When you test sciatica with a test magnet, you may get a reaction to both the south and north pole, or to neither.

Whenever Dr. Broeringmeyer treated sciatica he had to do double treatment. The south pole was needed to strengthen the muscle and the north pole was needed to relieve inflammation. So he designed a pad that would do both. He used alternating strips of north and south pole magnetic energy. This works because the magnet creates an arc between the north pole line and south pole line, which affects both the muscle and inflammation.

At the time Dr. Broeringmeyer first did his work with alternating magnetic poles, the best he could do was develop a pad with a strength of only 125 gauss, which limited its effectiveness. Later, he was able to design a pad with 3,000 gauss in each line. Since it had both the north and south pole, Dr. Broeringmeyer called his pad a *bipolar therapy pad*. Today, it's called a *biomagnetic therapy pad*. It is available from The Cutting

Edge and highly recommended for pain. It's also relatively inexpensive compared to the competing magnets on the market.

How the Bipolar Magnetic Lines Relieve Pain

The secret of the magnet with both north and south poles is the arc. The south pole moves hydrogen ions in and oxygen out. It vasodilates. It stimulates. It makes things acid. It gets rid of fluid in swollen tissue.

The north pole moves hydrogen ions out and oxygen in. It draws fluid to it. It vasoconstricts. Working together in the biomagnetic therapy pad, on sciatica and similar types of pain, the two poles combine to both stimulate and strengthen tissue. The pad is excellent for reducing nerve inflammation and repairing weak tissue.

Chronic nerve pain often responds best to the combination of north and south pole of the biomagnetic therapy pad. Used where there is chronic nerve soreness that is difficult to alleviate, it will often be very helpful.

Chapter Overview

Cancer

- We immediately use two 2 by 4 3,700 gauss north pole correcting magnets on the cancer
- We immediately use the correct PMG
- Put the south pole of the super magnet on the thymus
- Use standard process thymex and immuplex to further stimulate the thymus
- Use Super EFF to restore the phospholipid wrapping on the minerals
- Balance the bioenergy of the spleen
- Correct a south pole liver
- Balance pancreas and kidneys

- Use 3 homeopathic remedies: viscum album, vitis vinifera, and tuberculinum
- Use pancreatic enzymes
- Use mycosurge
- Monitor the adrenals to help deal with stress
- Eat an anti-cancer diet
- Use BTA and kidney testing to monitor PR

Heart Disease

- Use Cataplex B and/or Cardio-Plus to get vitamin B_4
- Cataplex B can help arrythmia, murmur and heart enlargement
- Vitamin E_2 is recommended for all people with heart problems who do physical work
- Cataplex G and Folic Acid B_{12} can prevent excess homocysteine
- Cataplex F can restore proper heart sounds and energy (add calcium lactate as needed)
- Cataplex C and Cataplex E help the heart repair itself
- Use Cardio-Plus for heart problems with high blood pressure
- Use Vasculin with Cataplex F and Cataplex D for heart problems with low blood pressure
- To balance and maintain heart health we recommend a combination of Cardio-Plus, Cataplex B and Folic Acid B_{12}

Pain

- Most pain is south pole. For south pole pain use the magnetic north pole
- North pole attracts fluid. If put on a painful area with swelling it will increase the pain

- In pain that involves swelling a fluid, the fluid must be removed first by putting a north pole 1 to 2 inches away from the fluid or a south pole over the fluid

- Disc pain and back pain that is neutral (neither north or south pole) may respond to the magnetic north pole

- In pain that involves both inflammation and muscle weakness (like sciatica) an alternative pad using strips of both north and south poles (like the biomagnetic therapy pad) is needed

CHAPTER 15

You Do Not Have the Right to Be Sick!

The ultimate justification of life in earth, air and water is to be found always in the simple primeval happiness of the immediate experience of being alive.

—Llewelyn Powys, *Damnable Opinions*

Aside from the obvious, self-serving reasons for being healthy, if there is anyone in this world you love and/or anyone who loves you, there is no greater truth or responsibility than the following: *You do not have the right to be sick!*

When you get sick you create unhappiness not only in your own life but in the lives of those with whom you have any type of caring relationship. But, you protest, I don't choose to be ill! It's just something that happened to me. Something that I couldn't prevent.

But that's not true of most diseases today. Sure, there are illnesses that have a genetic basis. There are illnesses we don't even know the cause of. But most illnesses can be prevented if you take control of your health and do what you need to do. Let's face it. Excluding diseases with genetic roots and a few

231

other mysterious maladies, *you do not have the right to get sick!* By using the Biohealth System and the technology we'll discuss in this chapter, you can monitor and maintain your health so you don't have to get sick.

Every sickness has a pattern, an environment or a framework in which it occurs. Disease is a manifestation of the disease patterns within your body. You can choose the health pattern!

What Is Biological Terrain Assessment?

BTA is one of the most powerful tools for monitoring health in the history of medicine. It provides an incredibly effective way to monitor your health and gives you an amazing amount of information on your body. With BTA you know precisely how healthy you are right now. You will be able to monitor any health program you choose and *know* whether it is moving you toward health, doing nothing or moving you toward problems.

BTA has been tested repeatedly and has even been approved by the FDA. When used in concert with the Biohealth System, you can get stunning results.

BTA came into existence through the research of Dr. Louis Claude Vincent. He was hired by the French government to see if he could find out why different cities in France had such grossly different amounts of cancer. A hydrologist, which is basically a physicist specializing in water, Vincent set out to find what factors might be responsible for this.

Dr. Vincent discovered a high correlation between cancer and the quality of water a city drank. Being a physicist, the qualities of the water Vincent looked at came from the field of physics. He tested the water's acidity and alkalinity. He tested how oxidized or reduced the water was, which was basically measured by how many electrons the water contained. He tested the conductivity of the water and its micro wattage. Ultimately, he found that specific readings in these areas corresponded with health and disease.

In much the same manner as Dr. Broeringmeyer, Dr. Vincent found that disease and health were both processes. They didn't just happen out of the blue. They were an expression of patterns of electrical activity found within each person.

When a specific pattern was present, it produced health. When other patterns were present, they produced disease. The farther a pattern was from the health pattern, the more serious the disease it produced.

Vincent's original research was on water and his conclusions are hard to dismiss. Since your body is mostly water, after all, it makes sense that the quality of the water you drink contributes significantly to health.

Vincent later extended his research further. Your body has three primary fluids in it: blood, lymph and urine. He wondered if similar measurements of these fluids would also tell you how healthy your body was. The answer was a resounding *yes*.

To measure the lymph it was found that you could use saliva and, not only did saliva tell you what was happening with the lymph, it also told you how effectively your digestive system was working. The real miracle occurred with blood. With the new BTA unit, it was found that *blood could be measured without drawing blood!*

The BTA Evaluation

For a BTA evaluation, all that is necessary is for you to bring in your first morning urine. At that time, you also give saliva. In a few minutes, you'll have a complete BTA evaluation.

The blood, urine and saliva each give three readings. From these nine readings a person gets an in-depth picture of his or her health. The greater the difference between the ideal BTA reading and the reading you get, the more severe the sickness that may be produced.

The BTA tells you exactly how healthy you are. Assume, for our purposes, that your readings aren't ideal and you do something to improve them. If what you did improves your health, at your next BTA reading you will register improved. If what you did made things worse, your next BTA readings will be worse. If it did nothing, your next BTA readings will be the same.

In his book *Prostate Health in 90 Days*, Larry Clapp devotes an entire chapter to how he monitored his cancer with the BTA. The title of that chapter is "Let Science Show You What's Really Going on Inside Your Body: The BTA Test."

I personally do not see how anyone with cancer would not insist on monitoring it with the BTA!"

When you're working with any health professional, it is important for you to take control of your own health and be an active participant in any treatment. With the BTA, you will know exactly how any treatment you're receiving and doing is affecting your health.

It is certainly possible, for instance, that a treatment will relieve symptoms and make you feel better but not improve your health. If, when you take your next BTA reading, the numbers are worse you'll know you're not getting or doing what you need. Although your symptoms are better, your body may be preparing to produce an even more severe illness. The BTA lets you know.

Once you start the Biohealth System or any other program, the BTA is a wonderful way to monitor it. With the BTA there is no guessing. Between the magnetic readings and BTA you will know exactly what is going on with your body. The BTA adds power, confidence and security to the Biohealth System. Whatever health program you use, for the sake of your life and health, we urge you to monitor it with BTA where possible. Your life and health are far too important to be left to chance. Don't take anyone's word for it. Always *test any results*.

To learn more about BTA, check the information at the end of this book. Apex Energetics has an excellent videotape on the BTA. (Apex also has a videotape titled *The Integra Terrain System*, which is a number of simple health tests you can have your doctor do or you can do in your own home.) BTA equipment is expensive and you'll need a professional to give and interpret the tests. Unfortunately, there aren't as many BTA practitioners around as we'd like to see, so you may have a hard time finding one. The BTA listed in the back of this book can refer you to the nearest practitioner.

The Isorobic Exercise Program

We have said that exercise is a great help to creating health. What is the proper way to exercise? Obviously, as with everything else, proper exercise is that exercise that is proper for you. But is there an exercise program designed individually for each of us? A program that will give each of us precisely what we need?

That is exactly what the Isorobic Program is and does. It is adapted to and for each individual. With Isorobics, you get a program designed by you and for you alone.

The Isorobic Program was first developed by NASA. There was a need to design an exercise program for the Apollo astronauts that would produce the highest level of health in the least amount of space and time. The instrument they designed was called the Apollo Exerciser. Today, that instrument is called the Isorobic Exerciser.

For Biohealth, you have three exercise needs—1) aerobics, 2) muscle building and strengthening and 3) flexibility. Filling one of these needs is not enough. You must achieve all three. No short-cuts permitted. The Isorobic Exerciser fills all of these needs economically and efficiently, in a small space and small amount of time.

Although there are some people who will spend two or three hours exercising daily and love every minute of it, most of us can't. If you're like me, time is just too limited and valuable to do much more than 15 minutes a day. That's why I need to get the optimal effects of exercise in the least possible time.

Hence the Isorobic Program. It's done with a small unit that attaches to your door. All it requires, as far as space, is 10 feet in front of that door. The unit is portable. You can easily take it

235

with you when you travel. It's also inexpensive and lasts a lifetime (two very refreshing features in the exercise world).

The Isorobic Exerciser also prevents you from overdoing it. Many people who begin exercise programs don't realize what they're getting into. They don't realize that excessive exercise can have negative effects. (Please remember, as in all Biohealth activities, excessive is what is excessive for you. What's okay for one person may be too much for you.)

One such excessive effect involves cortisol. Lately there's been much research on cortisol, a hormone made by the adrenal gland. When you're under stress, the adrenals make more cortisol to help you cope with it. When you exercise, the adrenals produce cortisol as a response to the stress of the exercise. Through an efficient biofeedback system, your body controls the activity of your glands. When too much of a hormone is being produced, your body slows down the production of that hormone at the gland.

Overexercisizing causes your adrenal gland to produce an excess of cortisol in response to the excessive stress. When this happens, and research shows it commonly does, the adrenal gland produces little cortisol when the person stops exercising. A person ends up with an adrenal gland that doesn't produce enough cortisol to properly respond to the nonexercise stress in life. As a result, the only time a person feels good is when he or she exercises because that's the only time enough cortisol is produced. Exercising thus becomes addictive.

You don't have this kind of trouble with the Isorobic Program. You don't have to worry about overdoing it or underdoing it. It is a complete (muscle building/flexibility/aerobic) exercise program designed specifically to meet your needs.

Details on obtaining the Isorobics Exerciser and information on the system are provided at the end of the book.

Adjunctive Help and Treatments

Using the Biohealth System—obviously—does not mean you know everything or can't benefit from other health programs. Far from it. With the incredible new research and technologies appearing every day and our knowledge increasing all the time, there is no one technique or person who can claim to have it all. Cooperation, not competition, is the key word in today's best health programs. As Biohealth practitioners, we are always looking for other health practitioners who can add to our knowledge and success. Our purpose is to cooperate with all practitioners and methods that, by testing, we find can add to what we are doing. Our sole goal is to produce the best possible program for you.

I have mentioned Marco Pharma and Apex Energetics as two other suppliers of fine remedies. With your ability to test, you will find others. Use this new ability as a major tool in your road to health.

That's one of the great things about Biohealth. Not only does it give you a solid foundation for taking control of your own health and life. It also gives you a way to accurately determine which other programs can be of help to you. It makes you an active partner with your doctor and/or health professional. Rather than being a slave to your health you gain control of your health with the Biohealth System.

The road to wisdom is always under construction. Because of this, there is no end to it. It is a road we happily travel "until the end of days." I thank you for walking this wonderful road and sharing its marvelous journey with me.

In conclusion, here are some words from the poet Kahlil Gibran, which sum up all we have said:

Like you, I have been here since the beginning...
...And I shall be
until the end of days.
There is no ending to my existence.
For the human soul is but a part
of a burning torch...
...Which God separated from himself
at creation.
Thus my soul and your soul
are one...
...And we are one with God.

Why Take My One-Day Seminar?

On December 8, 1995, at University Hospital in Cleveland, Ohio, a biopsy of my prostate gland showed advanced cancer with metastasis. I was told it was terminal and with treatment I might get one year.

On April 6, 2000, at Cleveland Clinic a biopsy of my prostate gland showed no cancer. My prostate gland was completely, healthy!

Would you like to know how I turned my terminally cancerous prostate gland into a completely healthy one? By the end of this seminar you will know how.

I was a partner of the late, great Dr. Richard Broeringmeyer. For eight years he and I gave one-day seminars. The subject of the seminar was how you can give your body what it needs so that it can replace diseased tissue, including cancer, with healthy tissue.

When I was diagnosed with terminal prostate cancer I used the Biohealth Program that I and Dr. Broeringmeyer taught in our seminar. This cancer program is described in Chapter 14 of this book.

The one-day seminar is an interactive workshop. You pair up with a partner and do the steps necessary on each other to replace diseased organs, glands, or tissues with healthy organs, glands or tissues.

In the morning session of the seminar you are given the information you need to understand the program. In the afternoon session, step-by-step, you do the health program. What has made this program so successful is that you learn how to test and prove that each step is right for you personally. You do not guess, you *know* what is right for you.

Why take my one-day seminar? Because we have found it very difficult for anyone only reading about the Biohealth Program to understand it and believe it. But we have found it almost impossible for anyone experiencing it *not* to understand it and believe it. I strongly recommend this experience.

For information on existing seminars or to set up one please contact the author.

Dr. Sanford "Buddy" Frumker
1731 Wrenford Road • South Euclid, OH 44121
Phone and fax: 216-382-3317

APPENDIX A: **SUPPLIES**

Following is a list of companies that provide the supplies we discuss in the book. Obviously, there are many more places where you can find supplies and we are not recommending you buy from any specific company. These are just a few we know of. What is important is not where you buy but that you *test* what you buy to make sure it works for you.

Biological Technologies International, Inc.

P.O. Box 560
Payson, AZ 85547
(520) 474-4181
They carry the Biological Terrain Assessment (BTA) equipment and program.

The Cutting Edge

P.O. Box 5034
Southampton, NY 11969
(800) 497-9516 or (516) 287-3813 (New York metro)
www.cutcat.com
We have purchased test magnets, 4 x 2 ceramic 3,800 gauss correcting magnets and super magnets from this company. With each super magnet we also purchase a 0.985 round magnet to hold it in place. They make a wonderful team. All of the magnets we have mentioned can be purchased from The Cutting Edge. They also have many fine books for sale. Send for their catalog.

Dolisos America, Inc.

3014 Rigel Avenue
Las Vegas, NV 89102
(800) 365-4767

>This company is one of many that carry homeopathic remedies. Dolisos has all the ones we use.

Fitness Motivation Institute of America

5521 Scotts Valley Drive
Scotts Valley, CA 95066
(800) 538-7790
(408) 439-9898

>They carry the Isorobics exercise equipment and program.

Marco Pharma International USA

1857 N. 105ᵗʰ East Avenue
Tulsa, OK 74116
918-833-5060

>They sell the excellent German Biological Remedies, which can only be purchased through your health professional. For information about their products, visit their Web site at www.marcopharma.net.

Nu Biologics, Inc.

30 W. 100 Butterfield Road
Warrenville, IL 60555-1563
(800) 332-3130

>We get our pancreatic enzymes, Pan 10X, from this company. You should also order their catalog. They have many products, including MGN3 and CO Q10.

Standard Process, Inc.

P.O. Box 904
1200 W. Royal Lee Drive
Palmyra, WI 53156
(800) 848-5061

You usually cannot buy direct from Standard Process but you can ask them for a distributor or health professional near you who carries their products.

To purchase products from Standard Process, Marco Pharma International, or Apex, you can contact Health Associates or the author (see page vi). If you have any questions about the products, we will do our best to help you decide what to order and how to use it.

APPENDIX B: **HEALTH SERVICES**

The Price-Pottenger Nutrition Foundation

P.O. Box 2614
La Mesa, CA 91943-2614
(800) 366-3748

Joining this foundation and subscribing to their journal, *Health and Healing Wisdom*, is a must.

APPENDIX C: **READING LIST**

The main purpose of a bibliography is to impress the reader and validate what you've written. This is not a bibliography. As Dr. Hans Selye, one of my greatest heroes and one of the finest medical researchers of our time, said, "There is no bibliography that can validate what you've written."

The only way you can validate what we have said in this book is to prove it! Once you prove it to yourself, it is validated by the only person who counts—you. We insist that you believe nothing but validate and prove everything.

Dr. Selye suggested not using a bibliography but supplying a reading list. I agree. The list that follows is for your greater knowledge and understanding. To experience these books has been a great source of joy for me. I invite you to enjoy them, learn from them and then *test everything!*

REQUIRED READING (According to Sanford Frumker)

Becker, Robert O. *The Body Electric. Electromagnetism and the Foundation of Life.*

Broeringmeyer, Dr. Richard. *The Principles of Magnetic Therapy.*

Broeringmeyer, Dr. Richard and Dr. Mary. *Energy Therapy Training Manual.*

Burr, Harold Saxton. *Blueprint for Immortality. The Electric Patterns of Life.*

Davis, Albert Roy. *The Anatomy of Biomagnetism.*

Davis, Albert Roy and Rawls, Walter C. *Magnetism and Its Effects on the Living System.*

_____. *The Magnetic Effect.*

_____. *The Magnetic Blueprint of Life.*

(The Davis-Rawls books can be purchased from The Cutting Edge.)

Epstein, Samuel S. *The Politics of Cancer Revisited.*

(Great information on why we have so much cancer and how to avoid it.)

Fromm, Erich. *To Have or to Be?*

(A great book on the art and science of living your best and fullest, as are all the works of Dr. Fromm.)

Lee, Royal and Hanson, William A. *Protomorphology. The Principles of Cell Auto-Regulation.*

(This is very difficult reading but, if you take the time to do it, it's a magnificent experience. To buy or obtain a list of available Royal Lee books call (916) 392-9644.)

Russell, Peter. *Waking Up in Time.*

(While not dedicated to Biohealth per se, this book is required reading for surviving the twenty-first century!)

SOME ADDITIONAL EXCITING BOOKS RELATED TO BIOENERGY

Bansal, H. L. *Magnetic Cure for Common Diseases.*

_____. *Magneto Therapy Self-Help Book.*

Barnothy, Madeline. *Biological Effects of Magnetic Fields.*

Beasley, Victor. *Your Electro-Vibratory Body.*

Becker, Robert O. *Cross Currents. The Perils of Electropollution. The Promise of Electromedicine.*

Becker, Robert O. and Marino, Andrew A. *Electromagnetism & Life.*

Bengali, Neville S. *Magnet Therapy, Theory and Practice.*

Bhattacharya, A. K. *Healing by Magnets.*

Bland, Jeffrey S. *Improving Genetic Expression in the Prevention of the Diseases of Aging.*

(This is a functional medicine approach to anti-aging medicine and consists of audio tapes and a syllabus. Call (800) 245-9076 for more information.)

Callahan, Philip S. *Tuning into Nature. Solar Energy, Infrared Radiation and the Insect Communication System.*

_____. *Ancient Mysteries, Modern Visions. The Magnetic Life of Agriculture.*

_____. *Exploring the Spectrum.*

_____. *Paramagnetism.*

Copson, David A. *Informational Bioelectromagnetics.*

Goldbert, Burton (editor). *An Alternative Medicine Definitive Guide to Cancer.*

(Of special interest is Chapter 34, Energy Support Therapies.)

Goodheart, George J. *Applied Kinesiology.*

(This is just one of many good books on Applied Kinesiology.)

Gordon, Barbara. *Medical Magnets, Nature's Healing Energy.*

Hannemann, Holger. *Magnet Therapy. Balancing Your Body's Energy Flow for Self-Healing.*

Holzapfel, E., Crepon, P. and Philippe, C. *Magnet Therapy. How to Use the Healing Power of Magnetism.*

Lawrence, Ron and Rosch, Paul J. *Magnetic Therapy. The Pain Cure Alternative.*

Leonhardt, H. *Fundamentals of Electroacupuncture According to Voll.*

Marino, Andrew A. *Modern Bioelectricity.*

Nordenstrom, Bjorn E. W. *Biologically Closed Electric Circuits.*

Norris, Noel C. *The Book of Magnetic Healing and Treatments.*

Null, Gary. *Healing with Magnets.*

Payne, Buryl. *The Body Magnetic.*

_____. *Getting Started in Magnetic Therapy.*

Philpott, William H. *The Magnetic Health Quarterly.*

(Highly recommended..)

Philpott, William H. and Taplin, Sharon. *Biomagnetic Handbook. A Guide to Medical Magnets. The Energy Medicine of Tomorrow.*

(Dr. Philpott and I have our differences. He says not to use the south pole. We want you to use it whenever needed. He says magnets cure. We find that magnets create the biomagnetic field in which healing can occur but they do not cure per se. Dr. Philpott does no testing and we could not live without testing.

249

Still, this book has much good information. Dr. Philpott has done much for magnetism and has some fine products for sale. Worth contacting. Call (405) 390-1444.)

Popp, Fritz-Albert et al. (editors). *Electromagnetic Bio-Information.*

Pressman, A. S. *Electromagnetic Fields and Life.*

Rinker, Fred. *The Invisible Force.*

Robertson, Arthur L. *Magnetic Therapy. A New Age Health Alternative.*

Santwani, M. T. *The Art of Magnetic Healing.*

Schiegl, Heinz. *Healing Magnetism.*

Versendaal, D. A. *Contact Reflex Analysis.*

_____. *Alternative Management Strategies for Practitioners of CRA.*

_____. *Advanced Techniques and Protocols for Practitioners of CRA.*

Voll, Reinhold. *Topographic Positions of the Measurement Points in Electro-Acupuncture.*

(This is a three-volume set.)

Washnis, George J. and Hricak, Richard Z. *Discovery of Magnetic Health. A Health Care Alternative.*

Williamson, Samuel J. et al. (editors). *Biomagnetism. An Interdisciplinary Approach.*

(From the NATO ASI series.)

BOOKS ON BIODYNAMICS

Tomkins, Peter and Bird, Christopher. *The Secret Life of Plants.*

(Fascinating subject.)

_____. *Secrets of the Soil.*

BOOKS ON NUTRITION

D'Adamo, Peter J. *Eat Right 4 Your Type.*

Decava, Judith A. *The Real Truth about Vitamins and Antioxidants.*

_____. *Food Fundamentals.*

Fallon, Sally. *Nourishing Traditions.*

(This book is a must!)

250

Price-Pottenger Nutrition Foundation. *Health and Healing Wisdom.*
(Call (800) 366-3748 for more information on this journal.
Membership in this foundation is a must!)

BOOKS ABOUT INTERACTING WITH UNIVERSAL INTELLIGENCE

Frumker, Sanford. *Mind Map.*
(Available from Sanford Frumker at (216) 382-5137.)

Kaplan, Aryeh (translator). *Rabbi Nachman's Stories.*
(Outstanding insights into life. Available from the Breslov Research Institute at (914) 425-5898.)

Steiner, Rudolf. *An Outline of Occult Science.*
(Every book by Steiner goes beyond being a book. It is an event, an experience, a step in your personal growth toward higher levels of being.)

Shepard, A. P. *Rudolf Steiner. Scientist of the Invisible.*
(A biography and wonderful discussion of Steiner's work and philosophy.)

Schwarz, Jack. *The Path of Action.*
_____. *Voluntary Controls.*
_____. *Human Energy Systems.*
(These three Schwarz books, plus others, are available from Aletheia H.E.A.R.T. Institute in Mendocino, CA at (707) 937-0602. I have studied with Jack for many years, and in my life I have no greater hero.)

GENERAL INTEREST

Sowell, Thomas. *The Vision of the Anointed.*
(In my biased opinion, this is a very important book and a great help in understanding the problems, disagreements and controversy we're having in the health field today. It provides wonderful information that will help you map your path to health.)

THE ART OF LIVING

Osbon, Diane K. *A Joseph Campbell Companion.*
(A wonderful introduction to living your bliss.)

251

INDEX

A

Adjunctive treatments 237
Adrenal glands 138–139
Alcoholism 198
Allergy 198–199
Anderson, Mark 183
Anemia 198–199
Apex Energetics 237
Arrhythmia 217–218
Atom 48–50, 91-92
  Hiroshima 49
Autoimmune attack 171–174

B

B_1 216–217
B_4 216–217
Balanced bioenergy 118–119
Becker, Dr. Robert 28
  The Body Electric—Electro-
    magnetism and the Founda-
    tion of Life 28
Big Bang Theory 46–47
Bioenergy 20, 24–25
Biohealth 199–203
  summary 199–203
Biohealth program 9–10,
  187–191
  applying 187–188

  definition of 9–10
  monitoring 187–188
Biohealth system 31–33,
  71–77, 158
  advantages of 32–33
  seven-step 71–77
  summary of 31–32
Biological health 188–191
  maintaining correct function
    190–191
  proving 188–190
Biological Terrain Assessment
  (BTA) 213, 232–235
Blood 147–148
Body electric 27–28
Bowel disorders 198–199
Broeringmeyer, Dr. Richard
  1–5, 100, 158–159,
  196-199, 204
Burr, Dr. Harold Saxton
  61, 64.
  See also Hunt, E. K.
Burr, Harold Saxton 66

C

Cancer 204–214, 227–228
  CO Q10 211
  failures 214

healthy food 212–213
homeopathic remedies 207
liver 208
Marco Pharma 211
metabolism 211–212
MGN3 211
minerals 206–207
monitoring 213–214
Mycosurge 211
north pole magnetic energy 204–206
overview 227
pancreas 207–208
protomophogen 206
spleen 210
thymus 209
thyroid 210–211
Tuberculinum 100C 211
Cataplex G, C and E 221–223
Cell disease 98–100
Dr. Broeringmeyer, Richard 100
Central nervous system (CNS) 116
Clapp, Larry 234
Prostate Health in 90 Days 234
Clorox 194
Colon 144–145

D

Davis, Albert Roy 36, 82-84, 158
Diabetes mellitus 198–199
Disease patterns 196–197
Diverticulitis 145
Dolly the sheep 36

E

Einstein, Albert 59, 103

Energy-balancing magnet 159–162
types 159–162
understanding 159
Epilepsy 198–199
Essence 28–30
definition of 28

F

Food testing 179–180
Frumker, Sanford C. 77
Functional energy 94–96

G

Gall bladder 138
Genetics 34–38
Gibran, Kahlil 237
Glands 137

H

Health myths 12–21
Heart 146–147
Heart disease 215–216, 228
overview 228
Heart enlargement 218–219
Hiatal hernia 142
High blood pressure/hypertension 198–199
Hoffer, Eric 77
Homocysteine 220–221
Hunt, E. K. 61–64.
See also Burr, Harold Saxton
Blueprint for Immortality 62–64
professor of anatomy emeritus at Yale 61–64
Hydrogen ion 92–96
pH (potential hydrogen) 93–96

Hypertension
  See High blood pressure
Hypotension
  See Low blood pressure

I
Information substance.
  See Stonier, Dr. Tom: IS
Inner teacher 39–41
Ionizable calcium 221–223
IS. *See* Stonier, Tom:
  information substance
Isorobic exercise program
  235–236

K
Kidneys 139–140

L
Lederman, Leon 24
  The God Particle 24
Lee, Royal 171, 215, 217
  protomorphology 171–172
Liver 138
Low blood pressure/hypoten-
  sion 199
Lungs 147

M
Magnetic examination
  131–148
  basic 132–133
  bone identification markers
    134–135
  identification markers 133
  muscle identification mark-
    ers 135–192
  surface identification mark-
    ers 133

where and how to test
  137–148
Magnetism 79–89
  definition of 79
  effects on small animals
    84–86
  mice and rats 85–86
  effects on the living system
    82–83
  flow of 81
  magnetic field 80
Marco Pharma 237

N
NASA 235
Nobel Prize 211
North pole magnetic energy
  86–87
Nutrition 174–177

O
Occam's razor 30
Organelles 98
Organic homeopathics 174
Ovaries 143

P
Pain 224–227, 228–229
  overview 228–229
Pancreas 137
Parathyroid 140–141
Parcells, Hazel 181
Pesticides and chemicals 194
  removing from food
    194–196
pH. *See* Hydrogen ion: pH
  (potential hydrogen)
Pineal 146
Pituitary 145–146

PMG 74–77. *See also* protomorphogen
Popp, Dr. Fritz-Albert 50–51, 61, 64–67
biophotons 64
study of 50–51
Electromagnetic Bio-Information 65–67
Potential hydrogen. *See* Hydrogen Ion: pH
Powys, Llewelyn 1, 11, 23, 43, 57, 69, 79, 91, 97, 111, 131, 157, 203, 224, 231
A Pagan's Pilgrimage 57
Cradle of God, The 203
Damnable Opinions 131, 231
Glory of Life 111
Impassioned Clay 91, 97, 157
Now That The Gods Are Dead 11, 23, 79
Pathetic Fallacy, The 69
Skin for Skin 1, 43
Pregnant women 129
Prostate gland 143–144
Protomorphogens 74, 172-174, 186-187. *See also* PMG
testing 186–187

Q
Quarks 23–24

R
Ravitz, Dr. Leonard J. 63
Rawls, Walter C. 82–84
Remedy testing 178–179
example 178–179

Restoring balance 168–170
Reversed polarity 98
Right carotid artery 135–137

S
Schmitt, Dr. Francis 44
Massachusetts Institute of Technology 44
Scientific method 16–17
Sinusitis 199
South pole magnetic energy 88
Spleen 143
Standard Process supplements 182–186
Sternocleidomastoid muscle (SCM) 135–137
Stomach 141
Stonier, Dr. Tom 44-45, 46, 47
information substance 44–45
IS 44–45
Super magnet 163–165

T
Test magnet 112-129
advantage 124–126
emergency muscle reaction 116–117
knee testing 127–128
leg length 128–129
placement 119–120
procedure for observing arm muscle weakness 120–124
surrogate testing 126–127
Thermodynamics 59–61
Thymus 142

Thyroid 140
Total heart program
  223–224
Treatment 170–171
  length of 170–171

U

Universal intelligence 51–53
Urinary bladder 144
Uterus 143

V

Vitamin E2 219–220
Voll, Reinhold 175–176

W

Warburg, Otto 211
Williams, Dr. Roger J. 18–19
  Biochemical Individuality
    18–19, 175
  *Wonderful World Within You,
    The* 18–19

Give the Gift of

TEST AND GROW HEALTHY

How You Can Turn Your Body into a Health-Building Machine

to Your Friends and Colleagues

THIS BOOK CAN BE ORDERED THROUGH BOOKSTORES,
HEALTH FOOD STORES, AND THE CUTTING EDGE

❑ **YES**, I want _____ copies of *Test and Grow Healthy! How You Can Turn Your Body into a Health-Building Machine* at $16.95 each, plus $5 shipping per book. Canadian orders must be accompanied by a postal money order in U.S. funds. Allow 15 days for delivery.

My check or money order for $_____ is enclosed.

Please charge my ❑ Visa ❑ MasterCard

Name _____

Organization _____

Address _____

City/State/Zip _____

Phone _____

Card # _____

Exp. Date _____ Signature _____

Please make your check payable and return to:

The Cutting Edge
P.O. Box 5034
Southampton, NY 11969

Call your credit card order to: 800-497-9516 or 516-287-3813